Incivility Among Nursing Professionals in Clinical and Academic Environments:

Emerging Research and Opportunities

Cheryl Green
Southern Connecticut State University, USA

A volume in the Advances in Medical Technologies and Clinical Practice (AMTCP) Book Series

IGI Global
DISSEMINATOR OF KNOWLEDGE

Published in the United States of America by
IGI Global
Medical Information Science Reference (an imprint of IGI Global)
701 E. Chocolate Avenue
Hershey PA, USA 17033
Tel: 717-533-8845
Fax: 717-533-8661
E-mail: cust@igi-global.com
Web site: http://www.igi-global.com

Library of Congress Cataloging-in-Publication Data

Names: Green, Cheryl, 1968- author.
Title: Incivility among nursing professionals in clinical and academic environments : emerging research and opportunities / by Cheryl Green.
Description: Hershey PA : Medical Information Science Reference, [2019] | Includes bibliographical references.
Identifiers: LCCN 2018024785| ISBN 9781522573418 (hardcover) | ISBN 9781522573425 (ebook)
Subjects: | MESH: Nurses--psychology | Incivility | Interprofessional Relations | Bullying--prevention & control | Workplace Violence--prevention & control
Classification: LCC RT86 | NLM WY 87 | DDC 610.7306/9--dc23 LC record available at https://lccn.loc.gov/2018024785

This book is published in the IGI Global book series Advances in Medical Technologies and Clinical Practice (AMTCP) (ISSN: 2327-9354; eISSN: 2327-9370)

British Cataloguing in Publication Data
A Cataloguing in Publication record for this book is available from the British Library.

Advances in Medical Technologies and Clinical Practice (AMTCP) Book Series

ISSN:2327-9354
EISSN:2327-9370

Editors-in-Chief: Srikanta Patnaik, SOA University, India
Priti Das, S.C.B. Medical College, India

MISSION

Medical technological innovation continues to provide avenues of research for faster and safer diagnosis and treatments for patients. Practitioners must stay up to date with these latest advancements to provide the best care for nursing and clinical practices.

The **Advances in Medical Technologies and Clinical Practice (AMTCP) Book Series** brings together the most recent research on the latest technology used in areas of nursing informatics, clinical technology, biomedicine, diagnostic technologies, and more. Researchers, students, and practitioners in this field will benefit from this fundamental coverage on the use of technology in clinical practices.

COVERAGE

- Nutrition
- Nursing Informatics
- Telemedicine
- Medical Imaging
- Medical Informatics
- Clinical High-Performance Computing
- Diagnostic Technologies
- Clinical Data Mining
- Biometrics
- Clinical Studies

IGI Global is currently accepting manuscripts for publication within this series. To submit a proposal for a volume in this series, please contact our Acquisition Editors at Acquisitions@igi-global.com or visit: http://www.igi-global.com/publish/.

The Advances in Medical Technologies and Clinical Practice (AMTCP) Book Series (ISSN 2327-9354) is published by IGI Global, 701 E. Chocolate Avenue, Hershey, PA 17033-1240, USA, www.igi-global.com. This series is composed of titles available for purchase individually; each title is edited to be contextually exclusive from any other title within the series. For pricing and ordering information please visit http://www.igi-global.com/book-series/advances-medical-technologies-clinical-practice/73682. Postmaster: Send all address changes to above address.

Titles in this Series

For a list of additional titles in this series, please visit:
http://www.igi-global.com/book-series/advances-medical-technologies-clinical-practice/73682

Advanced Classification Techniques for Healthcare Analysis
Chinmay Chakraborty (Birla Institute of Technology Mesra, India)
Medical Information Science Reference • ©2019 • 424pp • H/C (ISBN: 9781522577966) • US $285.00

Tele-Audiology and the Optimization of Hearing Healthcare Delivery
Elaine Saunders (Blamey Saunders Hears, Australia)
Medical Information Science Reference • ©2019 • 274pp • H/C (ISBN: 9781522581918) • US $225.00

Design and Implementation of Healthcare Biometric Systems
Dakshina Ranjan Kisku (National Institute of Technology Durgapur, India) Phalguni Gupta (National Institute of Technical Teachers Training and Research, India) and Jamuna Kanta Sing (Jadavpur University, India)
Medical Information Science Reference • ©2019 • 300pp • H/C (ISBN: 9781522575252) • US $265.00

Computer Applications in Drug Discovery and Development
A. Puratchikody (Anna University, India) S. Lakshmana Prabu (Anna University, India) and A. Umamaheswari (Anna University, India)
Medical Information Science Reference • ©2019 • 332pp • H/C (ISBN: 9781522573265) • US $255.00

Computational Techniques for Dental Image Analysis
K. Kamalanand (Anna University, India) B. Thayumanavan (Sathyabama University Dental College and Hospital, India) and P. Mannar Jawahar (Anna University, India)
Medical Information Science Reference • ©2019 • 334pp • H/C (ISBN: 9781522562436) • US $225.00

For an entire list of titles in this series, please visit:
http://www.igi-global.com/book-series/advances-medical-technologies-clinical-practice/73682

IGI Global
DISSEMINATOR OF KNOWLEDGE

701 East Chocolate Avenue, Hershey, PA 17033, USA
Tel: 717-533-8845 x100 • Fax: 717-533-8661
E-Mail: cust@igi-global.com • www.igi-global.com

This book is dedicated to all nurses who strive to work hard, enjoy their patients, their students, and co-workers as they work to improve patients' health outcomes and educate future generations of nursing professionals. Incivility does not belong in the workplace and no nurse has to tolerate bullying. This book will assist administrators and nurse leaders within health care facilities and academia that may struggle to find resolution to incivility in their workplaces, to implement interventions that stimulate discussion about bullying, and solutions to end the problem. Nurses will learn not to tolerate bullying, support peers when nurse-to-nurse workplace incivility is witnessed, and adopt a zero tolerance to allow cultures of incivility to exist within the work environment.

Nursing is a caritas profession that requires people that enter into the profession to foster and develop relationships with others for the sole purpose of healing. Incivility within the health care environment is functionally, contradictory to nursing caritas. When nurses are educated regarding the effects of incivility on themselves, patients, and others in their workplaces, change is possible.

Table of Contents

Foreword

Incivility in clinical and academic settings is counterintuitive given that "caring" and "learning," respectively, are at the core of these industries and incivility is an uncaring and ignorant act. The incidence of incivility among health care professionals has proliferated dramatically in the past decade and is responsible for the loss of both employees and revenue in US hospitals. A 2016 report (NSI Nursing Solutions, Inc., 2016) documented that 17.2% of nurses left their positions because of workplace toxicity, costing hospitals between 5.2 and 8.1 million dollars annually. Among reasons cited by nurses for leaving their positions were verbal abuse and poor management, including incivility and bullying.

I spent a significant chunk of my career working with nurses to develop self-care and interpersonal strategies for use in difficult work situations. For example, in the early 1980's I was invited to "conduct an intervention" with an operating room nursing staff who, after months of verbal and physical abuse by a surgeon, had threatened to walk out. After hearing about the nearly unbearable insults, verbal abuse and the flying instruments which in a few cases had caused bodily harm, I asked the administrators present, including the Chief Nursing Officer committed to applying a remedy. I suggested a two-fold approach, a course of assertiveness training and stress management techniques for the staff and a directive to the offending surgeon to recruit and pay for his own circulating and scrub nurses. I learned over the years that problems of incivility and workplace toxicity had to be approached simultaneously from all angles; that sending messages to the targets of these negative behaviors was not enough. Aggressors also need to be understood, held to account and subjected to programs of change. The interventions worked for both the nurses and the surgeon, who was offered an economic incentive to change his ways. There are many facets to defining, identifying and treating problems of incivility among health professionals in clinical and academic environments. This book examines (1) the nature of incivility and how it manifests in work environments including workplace bullying and lateral violence; (2) the effects of chronic incivility on the health and mental health of individuals; (3) the personal suffering of individuals who are subjected to incivility and bullying; and (4) strategies for use by individuals and organizational leaders to create a culture of mutual respect and restructure work environments so that incivility is called out and stamped out.

The aging of the US population and the rise of chronic vs. acute disease has increased the demand for registered nurses and for faculty to prepare them. The retirement of baby boomers, increased demand for nurses and toxic work environments are ingredients in the recipe for a serious nursing shortage. The author of this book is actively contributing to the prevention of future nursing shortages by focusing on the creation of respectful work environments where nurses can care for patients and teach students unfettered by incivility.

Gloria F. Donnelly
Drexel University, USA

REFERENCES

Nursing Solutions, N. S. I. Inc. (2016). *National healthcare retention and RN staffing report*. Retrieved from https://www.nsinursing solutions.com

Preface

Incivility and bullying in the workplace within the nursing profession has recently become a topic of interest. However, nurses bullying nurses in the workplace has historically been a longstanding problem. The old adage of *nurses eat their young* has been whispered on clinical units and academic campuses for years by nurses. Deemed as a means of initiating new nurses to clinical settings by giving them the most complex patient cases and watching as they either survive or rise above the stress, senior nurses determined the worthiness of their younger counterparts being able to handle the nursing profession. In academic settings, new faculty, likewise tested by senior faculty, are given high credit loads and difficult courses in absence of adequate mentorship and support.

Ironically, a profession founded upon caritas has failed to care for its own. Shortages of nurses and the mass availability of nursing jobs, has been used to mask why nurses resign from positions in academia and clinical practice areas. Turnover intentions seldom investigated as to the involvement of uncivil conduct within the workplace, left cultures that permitted incivility, to remain unchanged. However, research now acknowledges that bullying and incivility in fact contribute to nurse resignations.

Chapter 1 will provide an overview of the terms *incivility* and *bullying*. Uncivil conduct will be examined through a case study involving a perpetrator to provide insight into how a bully thinks and reacts with regard to their own behavior. Chapter 2 explores the phenomenon of bullying and incivility in nursing in countries such as Israel, Turkey, and Australia. Uncivil conduct experienced by nursing students, faculty, administrators, clinical nurses, and clinical faculty are discussed through the examination of current issues in various workplace settings that nurses work within. Imbalances of workplace tranquility and disruption influence work-life balance, as nurses attempt to find ways to cope with bullying and incivility.

Chapter 3 introduces the Reporting of Uncivil Conduct Chain of Command to provide support and direction to nurses that are experiencing bullying by perpetrators in the workplace. Unresolved and persistent, uncivil conduct can result in health and mental health problems for affected nurses. Chapter 4 provides nurses with instructions on how to report uncivil conduct that is not resolving and seek action against the perpetrator when mediation is not an option.

Chapter 5 discusses strategies that nurses and organizations can implement, such as Team Strategies and Tools to Enhance Performance and Patient Safety (TeamSTEPPS). TeamSTEPPS is a curriculum that can be used to improve teamwork skills, communication, and build team collaboration. Chapter 6 provides nurses, nurse leaders, and organizations interventions to understand, confront, and eliminate bullying and incivility from the workplace.

It is now time for nurses to have a voice and hold themselves, their colleagues, and the organizations in which they are employed, accountable for not permitting cultures of bullying and incivility in the work environment. The American Nurses Association (ANA) upholds a zero tolerance for workplace incivility and bullying. Hence, given that the ANA is the professional organization that develops and encourages nurses to adhere to a code of ethics and conduct, as a profession we have violated the ANA stance consistently.

If you are a nurse that has tolerated bullying and incivility in the workplace, it ends now. Organizations that knowingly fail to address or protect nurses that are experiencing physical and emotional attacks on a consistent basis at work, are accountable to the repercussions of ignoring the problem. Toxic workplaces not only contribute to a reduction in work productivity, but in health care, place patients at risk for medical errors.

Health care innovation, evidenced-based practice, research, magnet status achievement, specialized credentialing, and high reliability organizational strategies are just some areas that health care organizations have implemented to address risks for errors and create cultures of safety. Further implementation is necessary in the development and maintenance of cultures of inclusion whereby toleration of bullying and incivility is not condoned. Unaddressed, like a deep wound exposed to the open air, incivility and bullying will continue to fester, infecting the profession of nursing.

Chapter 1
Incivility

ABSTRACT

Nursing professionals experiencing incivility and bullying within the workplace are affected physically and emotionally. The sole purpose of the healthcare environment is to provide therapeutic intervention to the ill. Nurses should not anticipate going to work within healthcare facilities to be harassed, disrespected, and threatened. Be it a nurse working within a clinical environment or employed as a nurse educator in an academic setting, incivility and bullying can cause harm. Chapter 1 will provide an overview of the terms incivility and bullying. Uncivil conduct will be examined through a case study involving a perpetrator to provide insight into how a bully thinks and reacts with regard to their own behavior.

WHY WRITE THIS BOOK?

The decision to write this book comes from over 29 years of nursing practice encountering incivility and bullying in the workplace in my roles as a direct care nurse, nurse educator, supervisor, consultant, and director. In my role as a licensed clinical social worker, I have also provided therapy and counseling to health care professionals that experienced incivility and bullying in the workplace. Nursing is a profession that women and men enter with the purpose of providing health care to others. Caritas is one of the driving factors for many persons who enter the profession.

DOI: 10.4018/978-1-5225-7341-8.ch001

The academic and clinical rigor that encompasses nursing training, focuses upon the five components of the nursing process; assessment, diagnosis, planning, implementation, and the evaluation of patients in the care of nurses (Alfaro, 2014; Taylor, Lillis, Lynn & LeMone, 2015). Foundationally, the nursing process for student nurses and nursing professionals, fosters the development of clinical reasoning, critical thinking, and clinical judgment (Alfaro-LeFevre, 2013). Application of higher level thinking in clinical practice by nursing professionals correlates with safer clinical environments and positive patient health outcomes (Quality and Safety Education for Nurses Competencies, 2019; American Nurses Association, 2015). Incivility and bullying behaviors can distract nurses and impede their ability to provide safe care to patients.

I am concerned that a profession founded upon the care of their fellow human beings, is being associated with poor behavior and unprofessional conduct in the workplace. Be it in academia, administration, or clinical environments, uncivil conduct must be addressed. When incivility and bullying is ignored and allowed to permeate within workplaces; everyone—patients, families, other health care professions, organizations, and nurses—are affected.

Everyone Falls Short

There is no perfect workplace because there are no perfect employees. Recognition of the finite mind(s) of self and others, helps to understand the human condition and why imperfection will always exist. However, how we cope and communicate within the workplace is an effective means of discussing the subject of incivility and how employees and employers can develop workplace environments that are healthy.

Effective Communication

Let's begin by examining the basics of communication, of which I will refer to as, *Communication 101*. Communication is a process by which verbal and non-verbal cues are relayed using a pattern of sending and receiving of information from two or more people. Communication can be deemed effective, when the sender of information and receiver have a clear understanding of the intended message (Berlo, 1960). Therefore, it is imperative that messages be clear, concise, and be explained in a way that uses language and physical gestures that are comprehended by both parties.

Communication effectiveness can be impacted by cultural differences, perception, hearing impairments, auditory processing issues, and undesired haptics (touch). Traditionally, open-ended and close-ended questions are discussed in communication techniques because in particular with interviewing, content should be free flowing with one avoiding yes and no answers that can limit conversational content. It is important for active-listening (being attentive and present) to be paramount in verbal communication. Respectful, thoughtful, and attentive listening causes the other person to feel valued. And valuing a person validates their self-confidence and self-worth.

Nurses can potentially interact with people of different cultural and ethnic-racial backgrounds daily, especially within large hospitals located in metropolitan areas. Nurses therefore benefit professionally in having the ability to effectively and respectfully communicate with others. One might even say, that this is a necessary job responsibility, because nurses use communication to implement patient orders written by providers in the provision of care to patients. And in communicating with patients' family members, significant others, and other healthcare disciplines. Patient safety and environmental safety in health care settings, is largely contingent on nurses' communication (ANA, 2015).

The Toxic Workplace

When one uses the word toxic, it can imply something (or someone) being deadly, potentially fatal, or leading to bodily harm. Colligan and Higgins (2006) describe workplace stress as causing employees to experience changes in their mental and physical state when working in workplaces that pose a threat or appraised challenge to the employee. Factors identified as contributing to workplace stress are types of hours worked, role ambiguity, career development barriers, organizational climate, harassment, lack of autonomy, negative workload, isolation, difficult relationships with co-workers and administrators, managerial bullying, and a toxic work environment (Colligan & Higgins, 2006; Kinman & Jones, 2005). A toxic workplace therefore is a work environment that lends itself to the physical and emotional harm of others, because a level of dysfunction exists. Nurses working in this type of environment are at risk for becoming ill. So, how does a toxic work environment look? Let's examine the following descriptors below:

Toxic Workplace Environments

1. Workers align with bullies in hopes to be accepted or avoid conflict
2. Decisions are seldom made secondary to disputes of power and position
3. Alliances are shifted based on exchanges of perceived power or knowledge
4. The truth is seldom honored
5. Lying is commonly used to gain popularity and alignment with the current popular group or person
6. Dishonor is respected more than honor
7. There is a decrease in productivity and poor outcomes for the quality of work
8. Workers are stressed and may call-out ill frequently related to illness
9. Workers are symptomatic with headaches, gastrointestinal symptoms, and anxiety
10. There is a turnover of staff at least every one to three years
11. Workers belittle one another or speak rudely of one another's ability to perform their job

Alone With the Problem

When a nurse is being bullied, it is normal to feel isolated and alone. These feelings of isolation and loneliness are what the bully desires the affected person to have. Bullies exert power and control over their victims by weakening their defenses. Weakened defenses are manifested by the victim who becomes more quiet and withdrawn, experiences a decrease in work productivity, and becomes emotionally fragile.

It is important that victims not allow the bully or bullies to gain or maintain power and control over them. Victims of bullying can accomplish this by sharing their story privately with a trusted person. By telling another person about their situation at work and the bullying being experienced, victims minimize their isolation and loneliness in coping with the workplace incivility. The victim can seek support and validation of their bullying experience from their confidant, which can be beneficial in the avoidance of the tendency to blame one's self for being a victim or being chosen by the bully because of a perceived personality defect or low self-esteem.

The Anger I Feel

It is not unusual for nurses who are experiencing bullying in the workplace to feel angry because they have done nothing wrong to provoke the uncivil behaviors. Affected nurses must realize that there is no consistent correlation with being bullied and discord between colleagues. Victimization can occur in absence of interpersonal conflicts. Hastening to harbor anger is what can become problematic for bullied nurses.

When nurses, take the anger they feel toward the bully or bullies and internalize it, this can make the nurse more vulnerable to mood lability, depression, and illness. For example, the affected nurse whom is normally calm at home in interactions with family, may gradually become argumentative and demeaning to family members. Anger, left unresolved, will fester, much like a wound unclean and left to heal in the open air.

Resolution of the anger can occur when affected nurses recognize that while their situation and what at they are feeling is not fair, their situation can be changed. The key is to apply self-care interventions that foster peace and contemplation as to why the anger persists. Self-care interventions can include: journaling by writing about the experience and reading aloud what has been written to oneself, to a counselor/therapist, or close confidant. Or, by talking to a peer in confidence about the anger that is being felt secondary to the bullying. Ultimately, anger is an emotion that can be controlled. Victims must learn to constructively express their anger, while not allowing the emotion of anger to overtake their lives.

Cowering in Silence

The bullied nurse is not obliged to cower in silence by anyone. Nurses that are experiencing bullying may be coerced by peers, a supervisor (or department chair if in academia), director (or dean if in academia), or Human Resources to not report the dysfunction of a perpetrator(s) at the unit or department (school or college) level. Appearance of dysfunction such as bullying within the workplace, is indicative of deeper more pervasive problems. Hence, changes may need to occur in the workplace such as the addressing of poor leadership.

The historical presence of, or new problem with bullying within a unit or department (school or college), is not the fault of the nurse that is presently experiencing uncivil behaviors within the workplace. Nurses are hired to perform job responsibilities, based on the category of and specialty area of employment. Nurses are not hired to be treated unfairly by others because of their age, gender, race, ethnicity, culture, or religious affiliation (United States Equal Employment Opportunity Commission, 2019). Additionally, everyone in the workplace is accountable for ensuring that a culture of safety and respect exists (ANA, 2015).

So nurses affected by bullying, need not cower. Instead, by following a respectful pattern of reporting of the uncivil conduct, nurses can help facilitate changes in their workplace and create healthy work environments. Reporting incivility per the organizational hierarchy, is recommended. It is important for nurses to remember, that to maintain silence is detrimental to their health, their colleagues, their patients, and the organization itself.

The Lie of Sorry

Perpetrators of uncivil behavior within the workplace, can have periods of what appears to be remorse in their interactions with victims. It is important for victims of bullying to be aware that the appearance of remorse is not always based on truth. Bullies can use, what I will refer to as *the lie of sorry, to* engage the victim and mislead others in the workplace that their relationship with the victim is supportive and any conflict has been resolved.

It is not unusual for victims to believe the *lie of sorry* and not proceed with making a formal complaint against the bully or bullies for their uncivil conduct perpetrated against them. While forgiveness is important, the addressing of the uncivil conduct is just as important. So toleration of negative behaviors does not become a part of the workplace culture, be it intermittent or long-term in its existence, incivility must be addressed. Remember, a truely redemptive heart seeks forgiveness and says sorry in private, with no one else around.

Restoring What Seems Lost—Me

Nurses that experience bullying feel hindered in the ability to be their true selves within the work environment. For example, the friendly nurse who naturally enjoys laughter, smiling, and celebrating the accomplishments of others, may receive feedback from the bully or bullies, that "no one likes them" and that their desire to maintain unity among staff on the unit is "useless and stupid." The affected nurse will begin to believe the statements made by the bully or bullies and withdraw, becoming quieter and not engaging others in conversation and purposefully making every effort not to seem happy or content.

As affected nurses change their normal behaviors based upon the negative feedback of bullies, this empowers the bullies and disempowers the nurses. It is important that nurses hear what the bullies say, but not lose their own identity in hope to resolve the perceived conflict they have with the bully. Nurses must realize that bullies challenge their character because of their own insecurities and often, envy of the characteristics that the victim(s) exhibit.

To change for another in absence of a desire to change for one's self, is not healthy. Self-worth is reflected when one can value how their own differences and beliefs make them unique and special. Never allow bullies to manipulate and confound the stable mind, to exert unhealthy power and control. Workplace bullying can be both physical and psychological. Bullying experienced within the workplace however, tends to be moreso psychological (Coolidge, DenBoer, & Segal, 2004; Nielsen, et al., 2015; Giorgi et al., 2016; Rodwell & Demir, 2012; Sauer & McCoy, 2016).

Heal Thyself

For nurses experiencing uncivil behavior in the workplace, the concept of healing and resolution of the pain of being targeted by bullies, does not readily occur. Nurses must seek ways in which to heal themselves. Be it taking a walk during a break, praying, meditating, or listening to music, some form of escapism from the bullying situation at work, is imperative.

Healing one's self can begin when affected nurses feel overwhelmed and unsupported at work. Whether these feelings are realistic, actual, or perceived, self-care must be started in order to protect the health of affected nurses. Learning to place a distance between one's self and the perpetrator by intentionally caring for oneself, is the beginning of the development of strength and fortitude to end the pattern of workplace bullying.

As caregivers for others, nurses' ability to self-care can be compromised. However, it is necessary for nurses to recognize the value in for example, going for a walk to clear one's thoughts, engaging in aerobic exercise to increase the heart rate, mindfulness, and mediating to reduce stress. Nurses who place care of the self in the forefront of their daily routine, will likely have the emotional reserve and physical stamina to endure and defeat attacks of incivility within the workplace (Green, 2018).

Incivility and Bullying

Civility in the workplace, according to Meires (2018), is a professional standard "synonymous with being courteous, respectful, well-mannered, accommodating, and gracious depending on the clinical context" (p. 95). Bullying and incivility, unlike civility, are psychological and physical threats that are intended to harm others. Nurses who bully other nurses are referred to as perpetrators. Perpetrators in nurse-to-nurse bullying, seek to intimidate those colleagues they deem as being intellectually a threat, emotionally and physically weak and vulnerable, or whom the perpetrators perceive have less work experience or knowledge of nursing than themselves.

Incivility is unprofessional conduct whereby the perpetrator is disrespectful, rude, angry and embittered in their communications with others. Behaviors associated with bullying are ignoring, assigning of heavy workloads, telling jokes at another's expense, belittling, intentional physical contact for the purpose of intimidation, repeated criticism in absence of inquiry, assuming of absence of knowledge, and verbal attempts to fabricate the truth for the sole purpose of discrediting another person. Sousa (2012) discussed how bullying can escalate to physical harm and threats that can include shoving, finger pointing, blocking exits as someone attempts to leave a room, and invasion of privacy.

According to Castronovo, Pullizzi, and Evans (2016) perpetrators may identify a nurse or a group of nurses to bully. A group of nurse perpetrators is referred to as a mob. Mobbing is a type of bullying that occurs in groups. Nurses participating in mobbing are usually attempting to exert power or seniority over another nurse or group of nurses. When mobs exist in workplaces, this is usually an indication that workplace incivility has been allowed to be present by leadership. Unfortunately, leadership may also be an active participant in the perpetuation of the bullying and incivility culture.

In discussing the relationship of incivility and role stress to workplace aggression, Taylor and Kluemper (2012), noted that, "The connection between a stressful workplace and dysfunctional employee is an important concern among organizations" (p. 316). Of concern is that stress can be experienced on a continuum and varies among employees based on life experiences, cultural background, coping skills and available familial and community support. Lachman (2014), in providing examples of disruptive behaviors within the clinical environment, noted exposing patients or staff to contaminated equipment or fluids, throwing objects, intentionally damaging equipment, and banging down the telephone receiver, to be occurrences exhibited by nursing staff. Perpetrators of uncivil behaviors may also gossip, engage in exclusionary behaviors for the purpose of isolating the receiver of the negative behaviors, share falsehoods, use profanity, name call, exhibit rudeness, verbal and physical attacks, slurs, and lack of support (Clark, 2013; Clark, Olender, Kenski, & Cardoni, 2013).

The Use of Case Studies

Fourteen case studies are present in this book. The characters within these case studies are fictional. The purpose of these case studies are to enhance understanding of the different ways in which nurses encounter incivility and bullying in the workplace.

Case Study 1 is hypothetical and the characters within this story are fictional. The purpose of this case study is to provide an example of incivility and bullying in the clinical setting involving Bob, a nurse who is the identified perpetrator.

Case Study 1: Bob

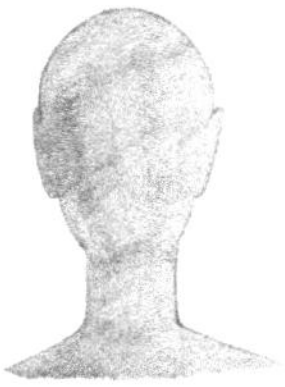

Bob became a nurse late in life. At 52-years-old, Bob was laid-off from his Wall Street job as a stockbroker. On busy night shifts on the medical unit, Bob could often be heard stating during report, "I am only doing this for the paycheck. Wall Street was a much easier and bigger gig." Bob had the reputation of not sharing the workload evenly when he was the charge nurse and would at times ignore the requests of nursing staff for assistance in transferring or repositioning patients complaining, "My back hurts, I will have to get one of those nurse assistants to help."

Nursing staff have repeatedly complained about Bob's behavior, but to no avail. Bob has a close relationship with the nurse manager and frequently works extra shifts on the schedule that would otherwise not be covered. Lately, Bob has been increasingly belligerent toward staff. He raises his voice on the unit, yells down the hallway to get the attention of other nurses, and questions the clinical practices of other nurses in front of their patients. Additionally, Bob always insists on being the charge nurse whenever he is working a shift.

The nursing staff is frustrated and four nurses have decided to resign. The nurse manger, concerned about the staff's complaints about Bob, meets with him to discuss his behavior. During the meeting Bob repeatedly says to the manager, "If it were not for me taking charge and covering shifts, this entire unit would go to pot! I make you look good to administration. After all I have done for you and this unit, and this is how I am treated! This is not fair and I can do better."

The nurse manager is shocked by Bob's behavior. He has only worked on the unit for two years as a new graduate nurse. The four nurses that resigned each had worked at the hospital for over 20 years. The nurse manager, as she listened to Bob's rantings, realized that she made a mistake in ignoring his unprofessional conduct on the unit. The nurse manager requested that Bob leave her office, then immediately called Human Resources to discuss disciplinary action.

Bob received both a verbal and written warning over the period of four weeks from his nurse manager, regarding his unprofessional conduct in the workplace and insubordination toward his manager. Angered by these disciplinary actions against him, Bob's behavior escalates further. He is more verbally abusive toward his co-workers and argumentative. A patient ambulating in the hallway observed Bob calling a younger nurse "stupid and incompetent." The younger nurse cried and was unable to be consoled. The patient, deeply troubled by what was observed, asked to speak to the nurse manager.

The nurse manager, after having spoken to the patient, called security and Human Resources, and in a private meeting with Bob in her office, asked him to leave the hospital property. Bob was escorted to his locker and requested to remove all of his personal effects. He was then escorted to his vehicle within the hospital garage and security informed him not to return to the hospital under any circumstances, until contacted by Human Resources. Bob quietly nodded his head and drove away, his head lowered in shame.

Examining Bob's Incivility

The person that exhibits incivility within the workplace is one that has often sustained a traumatic loss and deems the world as unforgiving and unfair. Multiple losses can be equated by the uncivil person, as grounds for mistrust of others and the necessity to guard themselves from others that they perceive do not represent genuineness, nor conform to their perceptions of personal and societal truths. Bob's loss of employment as a successful stockbroker on Wall Street within metropolitan New York, caused him to feel devalued and impacted both his self-esteem and self-worth. The necessity to retrain for another career for income and stability at age 52-years, was challenging and financially motivated.

Bob, unlike many of his nursing peers, likely does not view the profession of nursing as a vocation. Nursing to Bob, pays the bills. The emotional and spiritual disconnect from a profession that serves others' physical, emotional, and spiritual needs, can become problematic for nurses at all levels in their career; the novice and expert alike. Given Bob's verbal demeaning of the work of a nurse while on the job, he sees his former career as more prestigious. Hence, Bob feels angry and betrayed by his life's circumstances and lashes out on others as a means to exhibit power and self-validation, while attempting to secretly hide his insecurities.

Incivility has been defined as rude, disruptive, and discourteous behaviors and speech that are exhibited by the perpetrator(s) in an attempt to exude power and authority over another person. The need for power and authority may be related to an unresolved conflict, frustration, or insecurity (Andersson & Pearson, 1999; Feldman, 2001). Incivility can consist of verbal attacks, lack of collaboration, condescending language, sexual comments, blaming others, superficial listening, disregard for interdisciplinary input, withholding information, and rude comments (Felblinger, 2009). Other behaviors indicative of incivility are devaluing and distorting, misrepresenting and lying, shaming, splitting, breaking boundaries, excluding, betraying, and setting-up the victim of incivility (Heinrich, 2007; Peters, 2015).

While incivility can occur with physical contact, the perpetrator of incivility tends to use more covert activity to demean and emotionally harm victims. The disruptive behaviors that can occur with incivility, can cause physiological and psychological distress for the victim (Clark, 2013). For the person experiencing incivility, the public criticism, slurs, jokes and insults in absence of intervention by an outside party, or the victim seeking help, may progress into physical violence.

Bullying is the intentional disregard of another person with exacting malice. The difference between incivility and bullying is that incivility often consists of acts by perpetrators that can be observed by onlookers as being misdirected anger or frustration. Bullying is targeted behavior toward a specific person. With regards to horizontal/lateral violence, this constitutes both verbal and physical aggression. Horizontal/Lateral violence more commonly occurs within peer groups, hence, nurse-to-nurse incivility.

Bob exhibited bullying behaviors. He was rude and disrespectful toward his colleagues. His entitlement and insubordination toward his nurse manager revealed that he had minimal insight as to how his behaviors at work affected others. The latter includes the patient who observed Bob's behaviors, felt uncomfortable, and reported his observation to the nurse manager.

Witnessing Incivility

For persons or fellow employees observing incivility and bullying in the workplace they may feel awkward or helpless with intervening. However, within the profession of nursing, failure to act, provides permission for these behaviors to continue and can potentially harm not only the affected nurse, but patients being cared for by the nurse. The Joint Commission (TJC), is a non-profit, independent organization that accredits health care organizations nationally in the United States. As of 2018, TJC had accredited over 21,000 health care facilities. Organizations accredited by TJC are recognized within the health care industry, as providing quality, safe, and effective care to patients. TJC's mission and vision are:

- **Mission:** To continuously improve health care for the public, in collaboration with other stakeholders, by evaluating health care organizations and inspiring them to excel in providing safe and effective care of the highest quality and value.
- **Vision Statement:** All people always experience the safest, highest quality, best-value health care across all settings. (TJC, 2018)

TJC (2008) in addressing their stance on bullying and incivility within the workplace environment noted that disruptive and intimidating behaviors contribute to nurses resigning their positions, as well as contributing to medical errors, increased cost of care, poor patient outcomes, and poor patient satisfaction. Uncivil behaviors, can lead to hospitalized patients potentially having an increased length of stay because of medical errors. An example of a medical error related to incivility in the workplace, would be a patient receiving the wrong medication, because a nurse providing care to them was under emotional duress from being bullied within the workplace.

For nurses working with perpetrators of bullying, failure to report nurse-to-nurse incivility by a fellow nurse, manager, clinician, or administrator, can potentially lead to patient harm. Allowance of the workplace to become uncivil, desecrates the profession of nursing; as patients, families, students (i.e. nursing, medical, and other health care professions) and other health care professionals observe disruptive behaviors. The American Nurses Association (ANA) is the national organization for nurses that develops the code of ethics and standards for by which nurses practicing within the United States follow. In 2015, the ANA's Professional Issues Panel on Incivility, Bullying, and Workplace Violence created a statement of position for the ANA on behalf of nurses practicing within the United States. The ANA's stance on maintenance of respect and collegiality among nurses and persons the nurse interacts with in the workplace, addressed these key areas:

- The nursing profession will not tolerate violence of any kind from any source;
- Nurses and employers must collaborate to create a culture of respect;
- The adoption of evidence-based strategies that prevent and mitigate incivility, bullying, and workplace violence; and promote health, safety, and wellness and optimal outcomes in health care;
- The strategies employed are listed and categorized by primary, secondary, and tertiary prevention;
- The statement is relevant for all health care professionals and stakeholders, not exclusively to nurses. (ANA, 2018)

According to the ANA Code of Ethics for Nurses (2018), nurses are prohibited from fostering and/or engaging within the disruptive workplace behaviors of horizontal/lateral violence, incivility, and bullying. Intimidation and harassment within the workplace is not condoned. The fair treatment of others applying integrity and care, with commitment by nurses to resolve conflict, and adherence to respectful communication, is emphasized. Therefore, failure of nurses to report uncivil behavior in the workplace is a violation of their code of ethics.

A History of Victimization

Bullies have often been victims of bullying themselves. According to Reid, Holt, Bowman, Espelage, and Green (2016), children who experience bullying victimization, tend to become adults that have anxiety and depression. Children that have been bullied, are more likely to be resilient, when support is provided by family.

Uncivil conduct is deeply rooted in insecurity, frustration, and anger. Dissatisfaction with one's life can breed resentment and fear, as the perpetrator(s) seeks to redefine their existence. The workplace becomes a safe area, because unlike the home environment, it can potentially be an area where power and authority can be exuded.

Perpetrators of bullying tend to direct their aggressions toward others whom they perceive, may struggle to defend themselves (Gladden et al., 2013). The struggle that the victim of bullying has, is one of being "caught off guard" and in disbelief that the professional environment is so hostile. Also, the initial confusion as to why the bully or bullies has selectively decided to target them unprovoked by circumstance or a work-related interaction or event, seems illogical.

Perception versus Reality

It is important for persons being affected by bullying to realistically look inward and ask themselves, "Is there something about me (i.e. communication patterns or work patterns) that needs to be changed? Could I have done something that was misunderstood by the perpetrator(s)?" If the answer is "no" to these questions, then it is likely that the perpetrator(s) has targeted the affected nurse(s) without cause. If this is the case, then exploration is needed on the part of the affected nurse(s) as to whether the act of bullying can be resolved privately by meeting with the perpetrator(s) or is the mediation of a nurse manager or Human Resource representative indicated.

CHAPTER SUMMARIZATION

Historically, the first known documentation of incivility and bullying referencing the nursing profession occurred in 1909. An article was written in The New York Times describing how head nurses working within hospital settings were dictators who were abusive to the nurses they supervised (Castronovo, Pullizi, & Evans, 2016). Nurse researchers that have examined this article, believe that this may have been the origin of the phrase, *nurses eat their young* (Castronovo, et al., 2016; Meires, 2018). Regardless of the origins of bullying and incivility within the workplace, it has now become apparent, that these behaviors are unhealthy and impact the lives of affected nurses and the patients in their care.

Within Appendix 2 are exploratory exercises that address bullying and incivility. Please read each question and write your answer in the space provided. Discuss your answers within a small group of peers. If alone, review your responses and reflect upon your answers.

REFERENCES

Alfaro, R. (2014). *Applying nursing process: The foundation for clinical reasoning* (8th ed.). Philadelphia, PA: Wolters Kluwer Health/Lippincott William & Wilkins.

Alfaro-LeFevre, R. (2010). *Applying nursing process: A tool for critical thinking* (7th ed.). Philadelphia, PA: Wolters Kluwer Health/Lippincott William & Wilkins.

Alfaro-Levre, R. (2013). *Critical thinking, clinical reasoning, and clinical judgement: A Practical approach* (5th ed.). St. Louis, MO: Elsevier.

American Nurses Association. (2015). *Code of ethics for nurses with interpretive statements*. Silver Spring, MD: American Nurses Association.

American Nurses Association. (2018). *Violence, Incivility, and Bullying-Professional Issues Panel on Incivility, Bullying, and Workplace Incivility, 2015*. Retrieved from https://www.nursingworld.org/practice-policy/work-environment/violence-incivility-bullying/

Andersson, L. M., & Pearson, C. M. (1999). Tit for tat? The spiraling effect of incivility in the Workplace. *Academy of Management Review*, *24*(3), 452–471. doi:10.5465/amr.1999.2202131

Berlo, D. (1960). *The process of communication: An introduction to theory and practice*. New York, NY: Holt Rinehart, & Winston.

Castronovo, M. A., Pullizzi, A., & Evans, S. (2016). Nurse bullying: A review and a proposed solution. *Nursing Outlook*, *64*(3), 208–214. doi:10.1016/j.outlook.2015.11.008 PMID:26732552

Clark, C. M. (2013). National study on faculty-to-faculty incivility: Strategies to foster collegiality and civility. *Nurse Educator*, *38*(3), 98–102. doi:10.1097/NNE.0b013e31828dc1b2 PMID:23608907

Clark, C. M., Olender, L., Kenski, D., & Cardoni, C. (2013). Exploring and addressing faculty-to- faculty incivility: A national perspective and literature review. *The Journal of Nursing Education*, *52*(4), 211–218. doi:10.3928/01484834-20130319-01 PMID:23495699

Colligan, T. W., & Higgins, E. M. (2006). Workplace stress: Etiology and consequences. *Journal of Workplace Behavioral Health*, *21*(2), 89–97. doi:10.1300/J490v21n02_07

Coolidge, F. L., DenBoer, J. W., & Segal, D. L. (2004). Personality and neuropsychological correlates of bullying behavior. *Personality and Individual Differences*, *36*(7), 1559–1569. doi:10.1016/j.paid.2003.06.005

Felblinger, D. M. (2009). Bullying, Incivility, & Disruptive Behaviors in the Healthcare Setting: Identification, Impact, & Intervention. *Frontiers of Health Services Management*, *25*(4), 13–23. doi:10.1097/01974520-200904000-00003 PMID:19603687

Feldman, L. J. (2001). Classroom civility is another of our instructor responsibilities. *College Teaching*, *49*(4), 137–140. doi:10.1080/87567555.2001.10844595

Giorgi, G., Perminiene, M., Montani, F., Fiz-Perez, J., Mucci, N., & Arcangeli, G. (2016). Detrimental Effects of Workplace Bullying: Impediment of Self-Management Competence via Psychological Distress. *Frontiers in Psychology, 7*(60). Retrieved from https://www.ncbi.nlm.nih.gov/pmc/articles/PMC4753400/

Green, C. (2018). Understanding the complexities of the effects of incivility on the victim and using mindfulness to heal. *Journal of Health, Wellness, and Society*. doi:10.18848/2156-8960/CGP/v08i01/33-40

Heinrich, K. T. (2007). Joy stealing: 10 mean games faculty play and how to stop the gaming. *Nurse Educator*, *32*(1), 34–38. doi:10.1097/00006223-200701000-00010 PMID:17220766

Kinman, G., & Jones, F. (2005). Lay representations of workplace stress: What do people really mean when they say they are stressed? *Work and Stress*, *19*(2), 101–120. doi:10.1080/02678370500144831

Lachman, V. (2014). Ethical issues in the disruptive behaviors of incivility, bullying, and horizontal/lateral violence. *Medsurg Nursing*, *23*(1), 56–60. PMID:24707670

Nielsen, M. B., Nielsen, G. H., Notelaers, G., & Einarsen, S. (2015). Workplace Bullying & Suicidal Ideation: A # Wave Longitudinal Norwegian Study. *American Journal of Public Health*, *105*(11), e23–e28. doi:10.2105/AJPH.2015.302855 PMID:26378852

Quality & Safety Education for Nurses. (2019). *QSEN Competencies*. Retrieved from http://qsen.org/competencies/

Rodwell, J., & Demir, D. (2012). Oppression and exposure as differentiating predictors of types Of workplace violence for nurses. *Journal of Clinical Nursing*, *21*(15-16), 15–16. doi:10.1111/j.1365-2702.2012.04192.x PMID:22788563

Sauer, P. A., & McCoy, T. P. (2016). Nurse bullying: Impact on nurses' health. *Western Journal of Nursing*, *39*(12), 1533–1546. doi:10.1177/0193945916681278 PMID:27920345

Sousa, M.F. (2012). Management and Leadership: The elephant in the room- The truth about bullying in nursing. *Journal of Radiology Nursing, 31*(1), 29-31. doi..2012.01.002 doi:10.1016/j.jradnu

Taylor, C., Lillis, C., Lynn, P., & LeMone. (2015). *Fundamentals of nursing: The art and science of person-centered nursing care* (8th ed.). Philadelphia, PA: Wolters Kluwer Health/Lippincott William & Wilkins.

The Joint Commission. (2008). Behaviors that undermine a culture of safety. *Sentinel Event Alert, 40*, 1-3. Retrieved from https://www.jointcommission.org/assets/1/18/SEA_40.PDF

The Joint Commission. (2018). *About The Joint Commission*. Retrieved from https://www.jointcommission.org/about_us/about_the_joint_commission_main.aspx

United States Equal Employment Opportunity Commission. (2019). *Discrimination by type*. Retrieved from https://www.eeoc.gov/laws/types/index.cfm

APPENDIX 1

Figure 1. Blue boy

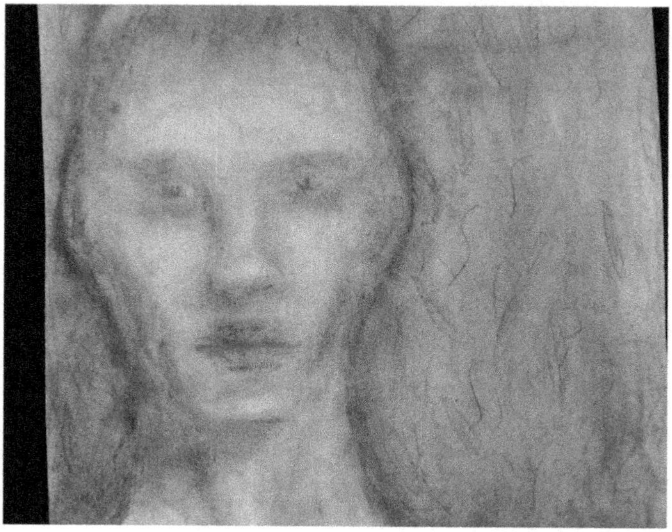

APPENDIX 2

Exploration Activities

Directions: The purpose of the *Exploration Activities* are to encourage reflection on the issue of uncivil conduct in nursing by recording one's feelings about the act of incivility.

What is your name? ______________________________________
Are you a victim or perpetrator of incivility?______________________________
When and where did your experience with the uncivil nurse-to-nurse behaviors begin?

____
____
____
____
____

What disruptive behaviors have you been exposed to by the perpetrator(s)?

If you are the perpetrator, why did you target this person?

Do you acknowledge that the American Nurses Association's Code of Ethics for Nurses does not condone the disruptive behaviors of horizontal/lateral violence, bullying, or incivility?

If you are a victim of incivility or bullying, what can you do to stop the perpetrator (i.e. talk to the perpetrator directly, notify your Nurse Manager, a Supervisor, Administration, or Human Resources)?

If you are the perpetrator, are you willing to seek help before you potentially lose your job because of your harassment and intimidation of a colleague(s)?

If you are the victim of incivility, have you considered leaving your current position? If yes, do you like the job and is it just the experience with incivility that is causing you to consider resigning?

What did you learn after reading this chapter?

Chapter 2
Workplace Bullying and Violence

ABSTRACT

Bullying in nursing is not a problem existing only in the United States. Nurses internationally are affected by workplace incivility and bullying. Chapter 2 explores the phenomenon of bullying and incivility in nursing in countries such as Israel, Turkey, and Australia. Uncivil conduct experienced by nursing students, faculty, administrators, clinical nurses, and clinical faculty are discussed through the examination of current issues in various workplace settings that nurses work within. Imbalances of workplace tranquility and disruption influence work-life balance, as nurses attempt to find ways to cope with bullying and incivility. The latter potentially leading to organizational issues with retention and turnover of nursing staff.

INTRODUCTION

According to Warner, Sommers, Zappa, & Thornlow (2016), workplace incivility is underreported and unrecognized. Trending of the incidence and prevalence of workplace incivility can be difficult. It can therefore be inferred, that many victims of incivility in nursing practice do not often seek help and suffer in silence. Lachman (2014) noted that "Incivility, bullying, and horizontal/lateral violence are examples of workplace mistreatment that injure individual nurses and the ethical climate of the organization. When these behaviors are allowed, nurse job satisfaction and even retention are affected" (p. 58).

DOI: 10.4018/978-1-5225-7341-8.ch002

Nurse Bullying Is International

Bullying and incivility in nursing is not a phenomenon limited to the United States. In studies conducted in Australia (61%, n= 762; Allen, Holland, & Reynolds, 2015), Greece (30.2%, n= 841; Karatza, Zyga, Tziaferi, & Panagiotis, 2016), Israel (29%, n= 156; Ganz et al., 2015), and Turkey (21.8%, n= 284; Bardakci & Gunussen, 2016) results ranged from 21.8% to 72.6% of nurses having reported experiencing bullying in the workplace. Etienne (2014) reported that 48% (n= 95) of nurses in the United States have experienced workplace bullying. As concern arises about bullying and incivility within the nursing profession, it is suspected that this percentage within the United States may be higher (Beecher & Visovsky, 2012; Wilson, Diedrich, Phelps, & Choi, 2011). Rainford et al. (2015) studied lateral violence (violence displaced on one's peers and not an adversary) within health care settings and found that approximately 97% of nurses have been targets of bullying within the workplace or have witnessed other nurses being bullied.

Incivility in the Clinical Nursing Environment

In the clinical settings, nurse-to-nurse incivility impacts the health and well-being of not only the affected nurse, but the patients in the nurse's care. Because nurses who experience incivility may feel devalued and question their own abilities, patients are placed at risk as the victimized nurse becomes ambivalent in executing sound clinical judgement and critical thinking (Peters 2014). The Joint Commission (TJC, 2008, 2018) and the Institute of Medicine (IOM, 2003) have identified the potential for medical errors for patients receiving health care in environments whereby bullying and uncivil conduct are tolerated; unprofessional relationships among health care workers and poor communication, impact the safety and outcomes for patients.

- **Tall Poppy Syndrome:** Tall poppy syndrome (Garland, 2018; Mancl & Pennington, 2011) is a term that describes a type of incivility and bullying whereby a competent, well-accomplished professional is criticized and verbally attacked by his or her colleagues. The perpetrators goal is to reduce the status of the person who demonstrates genuine merit and success in their career. The denigration of the targeted person is an attempt to discredit their successes and intelligence.

Within the nursing profession, an example of a nurse subjected to the tall poppy syndrome by colleagues is the nurse who is a whistleblower. A whistleblower is someone that is employed or was employed by an organization that reports a danger or wrongdoing occurring within the organization (Lachman, 2008). An example of a whistleblower would be a nurse working on a hospital unit that reports low staffing ratios affecting patient care to the Department of Health.

Incivility Within Academia

With low salaries (Wright & Hill, 2014) in comparison to their colleagues working within clinical practice, academic nurses must contend with the demands of balancing student advisement, teaching multiple courses, using current technologies in the classroom to engage students' learning processes (i.e. response systems, video, virtual simulation, and online examinations), research, and travel to disseminate research findings via presentations (Green, 2018a). Academic nurses also must be current in their practice depending on their institutions' requirements, and some nurses in academia may still work in the clinical setting via clinical rotations with students or in maintaining their own practice as advanced practice registered nurses. Nurses in academia also are more likely to bring their work home to correct students' assignments and enter grades into online grading portals.

Bullying behaviors in the academic setting occurring between faculty, can often present as covert. According to Dzurec, Kennison, and Albataineh (2014), faculty that are perpetrators of bullying, may use a subtle way in verbalizing to their victim, their displeasure with them. This subtle manner of communication used by bullying faculty, is meant solely to manipulate the victim's emotions and cause psychological harm by exerting power and coercion.

Heinrich (2007a) discussed the range of emotions experienced by victims of faculty-to-faculty incivility. The affected faculty reported feeling dismissed, having a decrease in confidence, feeling devalued, and disrespected. Faculty perpetrators of uncivil acts were cognizant of how their actions made their colleagues feel and verbalized a desire, to what Heinrich (2007b) refers to as, intentionally steal their (colleagues') joy.

- **New Faculty:** Peters (2014) conducted a hermeneutical phenomenological study with a participant sample of eight new nursing faculty. Faculty participants were employed within diploma, associate degree, bachelor degree, master of science in nursing, and doctor of philosophy programs. The new nurse faculty had on average, less than 5 years of teaching experience. The lived experiences of the new faculty was described, as these faculty struggled to remain in their positions while enduring the uncivil conduct of senior faculty, some of these senior faculty being their assigned mentors.

Qualitative narratives shared by the eight new nursing faculty were reviewed by Peters (2014) and separated into seven themes. These themes were: sensing that senior faculty feel threatened by novice faculty, sensing possessiveness of territory from senior faculty, feeling disbelief at the lack of professionalism, sensing a power struggle within the department of nursing, sensing others wanted new faculty to fail, and perceiving a lack of mentorship. The new faculty reported poor socialization to the faculty role with minimal support provided by senior faculty. The facilitation of open communication about collegiality and respect was suggested by Peters, as being beneficial in helping new faculty discuss uncivil conduct within the academic environment.

- **Nursing Academic Administrators:** LaSala, Wilson, and Sprunk (2016) conducted a phenomenological research study examining the lived experiences of academic nurse administrators that were bullied by faculty. The faculty bullying impacted administrators both professionally and personally. Emerging themes found in this study by LaSala, et al. (2016), were: the consequences of the faculty behavior on the administrator, the inappropriateness of faculty behaviors, and ultimately, the necessity of the nurse administrators to take action and confront the incivility and bullying within their department of nursing.

The LaSala, et al. (2016) study identified that bullying and incivility in the academic setting, when tolerated, affects nursing faculty at all levels in academia. Of concern is that when administrators are victims of bullying themselves, they are unable to protect or align with new faculty that are being subjected to faculty-to-faculty incivility. Hence, incivility and bullying can remain present within the academic workplace for several years in absence of intervention by affected nursing academic administrators. The latter lends itself to a toxic workplace environment.

- **Nursing Students:** Uncivil behaviors in academia have ethical implications. Nursing faculty provide the first example to nursing students of how a nurse interacts with colleagues, students, and patients (Burger, Malitas, Whitfield-Harris, 2014). Therefore, when nursing faculty role model bullying and incivility, nursing students may be more likely to accept these behaviors as being a norm within the nursing profession.

Nursing students themselves may experience bullying between nursing staff on the clinical unit. Unfortunately, nursing students can be targets of bullying themselves on their assigned clinical unit(s) (Anthony & Yastik, 2011) by nurses working on the unit(s). Incivility by faculty that is directed at nursing students can be difficult. Students have described faculty conduct toward them as being demeaning. For nursing students, the rigor of their academic work can prove stressful and anxiety provoking. So, when students experience disrespectful behaviors by faculty, their self-esteem, confidence, identity development as a nurse, learning, and self-efficacy are impacted (Del Prato, 2013; Backer-Condon, 2015).

- **Clinical Faculty:** Nursing faculty within the clinical setting with nursing students may feel overwhelmed with the number of students within their clinical group. The variation of student knowledge and ability to demonstrate the nursing process in practice, while applying the classroom theory with actual clinical practice, can be challenging for clinical faculty (Koharchik, 2018). With nursing shortages and complex medical and surgical patients that the clinical faculty overseeing nursing students is responsible to supervise, the job has become increasing demanding and can lend itself to faculty burnout. Faculty may become easily frustrated and inpatient with students.

Clinical faculty provided the opportunity to discuss student concerns and stressors encountered within the clinical setting with each other, clinical coordinators, and faculty, may feel more supported. Faculty provided the opportunity to contribute to changes in the clinical programs at their schools of nursing such as a decrease in student clinical paperwork, a change in a clinical unit, or reduction of numbers of students in a clinical group based on high patient acuity on a unit(s), will feel respected and valued. The latter can decrease burnout that may affect clinical faculty demonstrating incivility toward nursing students.

When nursing students report incivility and bullying in the clinical setting, their complaints should be investigated. Communication to students should be that there is a zero tolerance (ANA, 2015) for these behaviors in the nursing profession, no matter who is the perpetrator. In doing so and writing this professional responsibility within students' clinical evaluation documents, emphasis of the ANA code of ethics is made. Nurse educators will help to reinforce the importance of professional conduct in the workplace, clinical, laboratory, and classroom room settings for nursing students.

Faculty in academia that demonstrate uncivil behaviors are unfortunately, poor role models for nursing students. Students that are victims themselves of faculty incivility, can become angry, experience shame and doubt, become resentful, violent, stressed, withdrawn, distrustful, anxious, and exhibit hostility in their interactions (Altmiller, 2012; Thomas, 2018). Ultimately, students' ability to learn is affected (Thomas, 2018). These student behaviors, as a result, of the faculty (or clinical preceptor(s)) incivility, if unresolved, continue the pattern of bullying and lateral violence within the profession of nursing.

- **Student Nurses Who Bully Faculty:** Student-to-faculty bullying can occur in classes taught traditionally in a classroom setting and online. Online bullying can include arguments with faculty and students in discussion forums and rude written remarks or threats of harm. In the classroom, the student in front of others may question faculty knowledge of the subject matter; students may gossip to peers about the faculty, belittle the faculty or roll their eyes during conversations with the faculty. Student nurses who bully faculty can lead to faculty feeling frustrated and unappreciated in their positions. Faculty may begin to question their own competence and dread entering the classroom, online, or clinical environments whereby they must engage student nurses in learning. As a result, faculty can experience burnout and may decide to resign from their position as nurse educator (Meires, 2018a).

Student nurses may be unaware that their uncivil behaviors such as rudeness, belittling, and gossiping about a faculty person constitute incivility and bullying. Luparell (2011) noted that because nursing students are future nursing professionals, conversations about bullying behaviors help stop the pattern of incivility in the workplace. Nurse educators bullied by nursing students can bring to the students' awareness that their behavior is in violation of the ANA (2015) code of ethics. If the behaviors persist, faculty should notify their academic administrator and place the student on a progressive disciplinary action plan to improve their professional conduct.

- **Nursing Faculty Who Bully Colleagues and Students:** According to Meires (2018b), in academia, faculty bullies can be deans, clinical faculty, university administrators, members of an interprofessional team, department chairs, directors, instructors, and professors. Faculty may occasionally have days whereby they feel ill, fatigued or frustrated with their workload. As a result, they may be abrupt in their conversations with colleagues and students. These behaviors can become uncivil when the faculty member fails to provide self-care (Green, 2018a) by making time to eat, sleep, and rest. Thereby intensifying their own level of stress which is released by targeting others as the cause of their own personal disillusionment. Faculty who bully colleagues and students made aware of their behaviors must be held accountable for the correction of these behaviors in the workplace. Faculty bullying and incivility negatively affect the physical and emotional health of students and colleagues.

Case Study 2 is hypothetical and the characters within this story are fictional. The purpose of this case study is to provide an example of incivility in the clinical setting involving a student nurse and clinical faculty. Upon reading this case study, consider the value of prelicensure education on incivility and bullying in the workplace in the classroom and clinical settings.

Case Study 2: Bradley

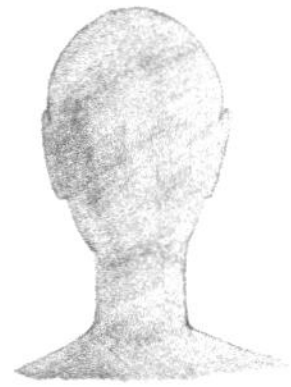

Bradley was a very engaging young man who on the clinical unit, is always kind to his patients and peers. A team player, Bradley frequently asks the nursing staff on the unit if they needed any help once his assigned work is completed. In the classroom setting, Bradley is a highly motivated student who strives to maintain at least a B+ in all of his courses.

Miss Joyce is Bradley's clinical faculty for his medical-surgical rotation. Bradley regularly goes by his clinical faculty's office at least once a week to review medical-surgical content during office hours, particularly when he has patients with multiple disease processes and poor prognoses. Bradley is sensitive and compassionate in the care of patients and always wants to improve his assessment and diagnostic skills in theory and clinical application.

One day Bradley visits the office of his clinical faculty. Bradley inquires, "Can I talk to you Miss Joyce about something?" Bradley shares being bullied by a member of the nursing faculty. Miss Joyce encourages him to go speak to the faculty member to share how he feels and see if resolution could occur. Bradley smirked and shook his head.

Miss Joyce again suggested Bradley speak with his professor reassuring him that she is an excellent nurse educator and would listen to his concerns. Bradley, usually calm and considerate, becomes frustrated and states, "Miss Joyce, the professor wanted me to write negative things about you. She tried to plant things in all of my clinical group's heads about undermining you. You might think she is nice, but she isn't Miss Joyce. She hates you and wants us (the students) to do the same."

Miss Joyce is silent. She apologizes to Bradley that a faculty member had placed this burden on him and his peers. Miss Joyce encourages Bradley to focus on his academic work and not worry about the situation, as she would handle it.

However, Bradley informs Miss Joyce that he had already spoke to the Associate Dean about the issue. Later that day, Miss Joyce receives a phone call from the Associate Dean who requests to meet with her. The professor who Bradley reported allegedly demonstrated uncivil conduct toward him, had attempted to falsify information about Miss Joyce.

Miss Joyce met with the Associate Dean, followed by the faculty member. The nursing student's concerns were validated. Disciplinary action was taken against the alleged professor and a letter was placed within the professor's file after several students shared with the Associate Dean how their professor encouraged them to discredit the clinical skills of their clinical faculty.

Unfortunately, Bradley was disillusioned by what he had experienced and contemplated leaving the nursing program. He stated, "If nurses that teach us treat each other badly for no good reason, and these are my role models… then how is the rest of this profession?" Miss Joyce and the Associate Dean provide support to Bradley and he eventually decides to remain in the nursing program and complete his degree.

Case Study 2 Questions to Consider

1. Why did the faculty member seek to discredit the clinical faculty colleague?
2. Does incivility and bullying affect future nursing practices of prelicensure students?

Case Study 3 is a hypothetical case study and all characters are fictional. The purpose of this case study is to provide an example of student-to faculty bullying. The site of the bullying is within the clinical environment and social media.

Case Study 3: Peggy

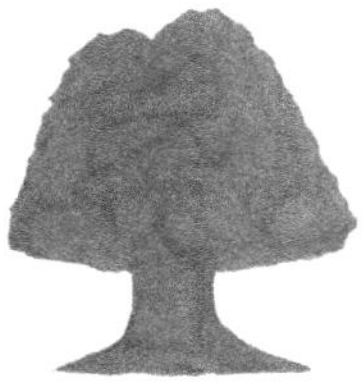

Lisa has been working as clinical faculty for a college nine years. The nursing students are wonderful to work with. The students renew Lisa's energy and faith in the nursing profession; she enjoys her work. Lisa's primary job is in the Emergency Department and she occasionally moonlights on the inpatient musculoskeletal unit.

The start of a new school year is an exciting time for Lisa and her students. She works with first year nursing students at the college, so each year she reviews health assessment skills the students learn in the classroom and nursing laboratory settings. Lisa also reviews and practices effective communication strategies with the nursing students, to use with patients, family members, healthcare providers, and other members of the health care team. Lisa frequently shares with her colleagues that it is a thrill for her to see the nursing students' progress as they struggle with auscultating an apical pulse, to eventually recognizing an abnormal heart rhythm.

Peggy was a nursing student in Lisa's group of seven students on a 22-bed inpatient musculoskeletal unit. Peggy seldom participated in pre or post conference discussions and seemed disengaged from her patients. Lisa, while rounding the clinical unit to observe the nursing students' progression with their assigned patient's care, noticed that Peggy's patient was tearful and lying in a disheveled bed. As Lisa walked closer to the bed to approach and speak to the patient, her nursing shoes landed in a puddle of urine on the floor. Peggy's patient, anticipating her arrival to assist her to the bathroom, attempted to leave the bed herself, but fearing she would fall, reentered the bed on her own just before becoming incontinent of urine on her hospital room floor.

Lisa provided the patient emotional support and immediately after searching the hallway, asked a nursing student to assist her in providing care to Peggy's patient. Once hygiene care was provided the nursing student and Lisa sat briefly with the patient and chatted. Lisa left the nursing student combing the patient's hair in the room. As Lisa completed her rounds on six of the seven nursing students, she saw Peggy returning to the unit with a male nurse. Peggy was holding a cup of coffee and flirting with the nurse.

After making eye contact with Peggy, Lisa approached her and asked to speak with her privately about her assigned morning patient hygiene care. Lisa shared with Peggy how she found her patient. Peggy explained, "I answered my patient's call bell and she was asleep when I got in the room, so I decided to go for a cup of coffee with the nurse Steve. Lisa inquired whether Peggy had informed the patient's primary nurse or patient care associate (PCA, nurse assistant) that she would be leaving the unit for a cup of coffee and Peggy stated, "Why would I do that. I was only gone for about five minutes anyway."

Lisa believed that Peggy was not telling the truth. Peggy seemed to have no insight as to how her actions compromised her patient's health and safety. Lisa requested that Peggy accompany her to provide a physical assessment for her patient and determine if she could help her patient with any immediate care needs.

Peggy rolled her eyes as she and Lisa walked to her patient's hospital room with both hands on her hip, and a smirk on her face. Lisa paused briefly as they approached the patient's room and reminded Peggy of the importance of professional behavior in the workplace. Lisa discreetly whispered, "Peggy, we all have days when we feel tired and even sometimes frustrated as nurses, but as professional nurses, we have to always remember why we are here---the patients are always are number one priority." Peggy stared at Lisa blankly and stated, "Sure."

When Lisa and Peggy walked into the patient's room, the patient immediately turned to Peggy and asked, "Why did you answer my call bell light, then turn it off and leave my room. I told you I had to go to the bathroom. You left me and I could not hold my urine. I wet the floor. I was hurt and embarrassed." Lisa was unaware of the full story until she heard what Lisa's patient shared.

Lisa apologized to the patient and so did Peggy. Lisa however, questioned the genuineness of Peggy's apology.

At the end of the clinical day, Lisa dismissed the clinical group and privately requested that Peggy stay and meet with her to discuss what had occurred during the clinical day. As Lisa and Peggy spoke, the nurse manager of the unit interrupted their conversation. The patient and the patient's primary nurse informed the nurse manager about what had happened under Peggy's care. The nurse manager said to Peggy, "This is an 83-year-old woman healing after a fall at home. You leave her unsupervised and having to use the bathroom to get coffee! She is a fall risk and emotionally, you have hurt her ability to trust all other nursing staff because you abandoned her after answering her call bell and doing nothing. I am very uncomfortable with you working on my unit young lady."

As an experienced health educator, Lisa is horrified that one of her students had intentionally neglected the needs of a patient. Lisa apologized to the nurse manager and provided verbal assurance that it would not happen again. She then completed her meeting with Peggy and informed her that she would be notifying her classroom professor, the Department Chair, and the Clinical Coordinator of her performance on the unit today. Lisa planned to meet with Peggy the following day at the college to review a corrective action plan to assist her in improving her nursing skills.

Professional Behaviors

Lisa reviewed with the Chair, Clinical Coordinator, and Peggy's classroom professor what had occurred in clinical. All parties were concerned about the patient's well-being and Peggy not having exhibited professional behaviors within the clinical environment. When Lisa met alone with Peggy, she too shared these concerns. Lisa inquired how she could assist Peggy in ensuring the development of these behaviors. Peggy simply stared at Lisa and stated, "I know what to do." She then signed the accountability/disciplinary action form agreeing that she would place the needs of her patients first and ensure a safe and supportive environment for patients in her care.

The following week, at clinical, Peggy was attentive to her assigned patient's needs and requested permission if she had to leave off the unit. All appeared to be going well. One of the nursing students approached Lisa and asked if she had seen a comment about her online. Lisa explained to the student that she was not on social media. The student asked if Lisa could accompany her briefly to the nurses' locker room so that she could retrieve her cell phone. The student then proceeded to show Lisa a social media post. Peggy had wrote how Lisa had humiliated her in front of a patient and yelled at her during a meeting at the college. Lisa thanked the student and assured the student that she would not disclose whom had shown her the post to her peer.

Lisa notified the Department Chair and Clinical Coordinator about the social media post she had seen online written by Peggy. The Chair and Clinical Coordinator advised Lisa to not discuss with Peggy about having seen the post and that they would speak to her themselves. Lisa concurred, preferring just to focus on assisting Peggy in meeting her clinical objectives in order to provide safe patient care.

One day while Lisa was working at her job within the Emergency Department, she received a phone call from the Dean of the School of Nursing informing her that she had been accused of yelling at her student Peggy within the clinical setting. Peggy alleged that Lisa made her so nervous that she was unable to do her work. Peggy had shared with the Dean that she had been receiving emotional support from a nurse on the unit; ironically, the same male nurse that she had left the unit with to have a cup of coffee. Lisa was devastated. She could not believe that this nursing student would not tell the truth, nor take responsibility for her own professional conduct. Lisa agreed to meet with the Dean and further discuss the incident.

Professional Integrity

Lisa met with the Dean and was informed that Peggy's father and mother had been to the college and shared that they were helping their daughter with applying for a restraining order to protect her daughter from Lisa. Peggy was being placed in another clinical group with a different instructor. Lisa was overwhelmed. The attacks on her character were getting too much to handle.

Lisa requested that the Dean allow an investigation to be performed by an independent party from the school. The Dean agreed. Lisa was instructed to make an appointment to be interviewed by the college's Diversity Officer. The Diversity Officer listened intently as Lisa shared the details of Peggy's management of the care of the patient on the inpatient unit. The final recommendation was for the coordinator of the undergraduate program to interview hospital staff and Lisa's clinical group regarding the alleged incident. Lisa requested to not return to the clinical unit during the investigation because she wanted the students and unit staff to maintain objectivity. She also felt too emotionally exhausted and distracted to work as a clinical instructor at this time.

After the Investigation

After the investigation was completed, Lisa was informed that she could return to work. She returned after two weeks and resumed the clinical rotation with her group. Peggy apparently repeated some of the behaviors in her new clinical group and received a clinical failure and dismissal from the nursing program because of integrity, professional conduct, and patient safety issues. As for Lisa, she is still healing. She is not the same clinical instructor. Lisa felt emotionally harmed by a student's incivility, her trust of others, impacted.

Workplace Tranquility and Disruption

Nurses, in absence of incivility in the workplace, are striving to achieve work-life balance within the ever changing healthcare environment (Green, 2018b). The necessity to remain current with technological innovations, new medications, and procedural changes, means the nurse is always in a state of learning. Tranquility in the workplace, is beneficial for nurses, because it enhances the ability to calmly apply critical and clinical thinking as care is being provided to patients.

Estimations of incivility in the United States within the profession of nursing, are that 27% to 97% of nurses experience incivility in the workplace (Beecher & Visovsky, 2012; Etienne, 2014; Rainford et al, 2015; Wilson, Diedrich, Phelps, & Choi, 2011). Mental health problems experienced by nurses affected by bullying include: depression, anxiety, heightened stress, decreased work performance, and panic attacks. Work-life balance can become an issue for nurses impacted by incivility, given the detrimental harm to the physical body with cardiac problems, tension headaches, neck and back pain, and gastrointestinal problems potentially developing.

Incivility contributes to turnover in the workplace and loss days of work (Cortina et al., 2001; Sauer & McCoy, 2018). Therefore incivility can impact the finances of affected organizations and departments. Nursing Solutions, Incorporated (NSI, 2016) is a company that works with nurses and health care companies for the purpose of securing employment within the health care industry. NSI developed a survey entitled, the *National Healthcare Retention Survey and Registered Nurse Staffing Report*. The NSI survey, was implemented within the United States and examined turnover rates of nurses. Survey findings were that registered nurse turnover rates rose from 16.4% in 2014 to 17.2% in 2015 for bedside nurses. On average, the cost for each nurse turnover ranged from $37,000 to $58,000. Hospitals within the United States, on average, can anticipate a loss of $5.2 to $8.1 million dollars. According to the NSI survey, for each percent change of registered nurses that leave their job at a hospital, the cost of these nurses departure is approximately $373,200 (NSI 2016). In academia, faculty shortages are impacted by nurse educator burnout secondary to academic workloads and low salaries (Wright & Hill, 2014).

American Nurses Association's Stance on Workplace Bullying

Within the *Code of Ethics for Nurses with Interpretive Statements*, the American Nurses Association under Provision 1 states, "The nurse practices with compassion and respect for the inherent dignity, worth, and unique attributes of every person" (ANA, 2015, p. 1). Standard 1.5 *Relationships with Colleagues and Others,* under Provision 1 addresses the expectation of nurses by the ANA, to be respectful in their professional interactions with their colleagues and all other people of whom they interface with in the workplace. Standard 1.5 is written below.

Relationships with Colleagues and Others

Respect for persons extends to all individuals with whom the nurse interacts. Nurses maintain professional, respectful, and caring relationships with colleagues and are committed to fair treatment, transparency, integrity-preserving compromise, and the best resolution of conflicts. Nurses function in many roles and settings, including direct care provider, care coordinator, administrator, educator, policy maker, researcher, and consultant.

The nurse creates an ethical environment and culture of civility and kindness, treating colleagues, coworkers, employees, students, and others with dignity and respect. This standard of conduct includes an affirmative duty to act to prevent harm. Disregard for the effects of one's actions on others, bullying, harassment, intimidation, manipulation, threats, or violence are always morally unacceptable behaviors. Nurses value the distinctive contribution of individuals or groups as they seek to achieve safe, quality patient outcomes in all settings. Additionally, they collaborate to meet the shared goals of providing compassionate, transparent, and effective health services. (ANA, 2015)

ANA standard 1.5 *Relationships with Colleagues and Others*, clearly explains the professional responsibility of nurses within the workplace, to exhibit civil conduct. The tolerance of incivility within the workplace by nurses, would therefore constitute noncompliance with this standard. Nurses' failure to follow this standard is a direct violation of their code of ethics.

Nurse and Patient Impact

According to The Joint Commission (TJC, 2016), workplace incivility in health care is on the rise. In 2012, TJC published, *Improving Patient and Worker Safety: Opportunities for* Synergy, *Collaboration, and Innovation.* This publication by TJC, emphasized the importance of maintaining cultures of safety within health care environments for health care workers, and the patients in their care. Uncivil conduct in the workplace was identified as a key culprit in undermining the health and safety of patients and persons providing care to them.

Over 50% (n= 3, 765, 2014 ANA Health Risk Appraisal Survey) of nurses and nursing students within a 12-month period of time, in the United States, reported being verbally abused within the health care environment and 21% were physically assaulted. Additionally, 12% of emergency department nurses (OSHA, 2016) were exposed to physical violence and 59% (n=7, 169, 2009-2011, Emergency Nurses Association Survey) of nurses were verbally abused within a 7-day period of time (OSHA, 2015).

In 2014, the Workplace Bullying Institute (WBI) completed a survey that examined patterns of uncivil conduct within workplace environments. The WBI survey found that female bullies targeted other females in 68% of cases and that males represented 69% of workplace bullies and targeted females 57% of the time. WBI reported that approximated 65.6 million workers within the United States have either witnessed or been directly impacted by bullying within the workplace (WBI, 2014).

The Institute of Medicine (IOM, 2003) report entitled, *Keeping Patients Safe: Transforming the Work Environment of Nurses*, brought attention to the fact that not only are nurses impacted psychologically and physiologically by uncivil behaviors within the workplace, but so are their patients. Patient safety can be compromised by nurses that are not able to focus or are emotionally distraught from being targeted by a bully, or bullies, in the workplace. Nursing is a job that requires nurses to both critically think, and clinically identify and treat complex diseases and conditions with medication administration, physical assessments, the use of innovative medical and surgical technologies, wound care, laboratory and diagnostics—all while collaborating with other disciplines (i.e. physicians, respiratory therapists, speech pathologists, dietary, psychiatry, social work, case managers, palliative care practitioners, environmental services, etc.) to ensure the stability and well-being of patients in their care. Potentially, medical errors can be made and patients' safety compromised, when uncivil behaviors are condoned in the workplace.

Protecting Your Patients and Your License

Nurses' course of academic studies to obtain their licensure(s) are rigorous. The combination of theory and clinical practice requirements occur simultaneously. Work-life balance for prelicensure nursing students, can be challenging. Therefore, when a graduate nurse obtains state licensure, this is a time of celebration, as their nursing journey begins. With this nursing journey is the honor to care for patients.

Because the focus of the profession is the providing of health education and direct care to the infirmed, nurses can initially be surprised or confused by acts of incivility in the workplace. It is imperative that nurses working in direct care with patients, especially, realize that uncivil conduct can impact their care of patients. Thereby, putting the patient at risk for an error by a nurse experiencing an impaired self-concept secondary to being bullied by a co-worker.

The duty of the nurse is to protect their patients. According to the ANA Code of Ethics for Nurses with Interpretive Statements (ANA, 2015) Provision 2, "The nurse's primary commitment is to the patient, whether an individual, family, group, community, or population" (ANA, 205, p. 5). Provision 2.1, the Primacy of the Patient's Interests, written below, addresses in more detail, the importance of nurses placing the interests of patients first, at all times.

The nurse's primary commitment is to the recipients of nursing and healthcare services—patient or client—whether individuals, families, groups, communities, or populations. Each plan of care must reflect the fundamental commitment of nursing to the uniqueness, worth, and dignity of the patient. Nurses provide patients with opportunities to participate in planning and implementing care and support that are acceptable to the patient. Honest discussions about available resources, treatment options, and capacity for self-care are essential. Addressing patient interests requires recognition of the patient's place within the family and other relationships. When the patient's wishes are in conflict with those of others, nurses help to resolve the conflict. Where conflict persists, the nurse's commitment remains to the identified patient. (ANA, 2015, p. 5)

It is imperative that nurses view incivility as being in conflict with their commitment to their identified patients. Failure of the nurse to address or bring to the attention of other nurses, administrators, Human Resource Departments, and managers, the uncivil behaviors of bullies within the health care environment, may potentially put patients' provision of health care in jeopardy and nurses' license(s) at risk if patient harm occurs. Because patient care delivery is the primary role of nurses, any disturbances or disruptions affecting nursing judgement, is unsafe for patients.

Within Appendix 2 are exploration activities to be completed privately or within a classroom setting for discussion.

REFERENCES

American Nurses Association. (2014). *American Nurses Association Health Risk Appraisal (HRA): Preliminary Findings October 2013–October 2014.* Academic Press.

American Nurses Association. (2015). Code of ethics for nurses with interpretive statements. Silver Spring, MA: Nursebooks.org.

Anthony, M. & Yastik, J. (2011). Nursing students' experiences with incivility in clinical education. *Journal of Nursing Education, 50*(10), 140-144. doi: 10.3928/01484834-20110131-4

Backer-Condon, B. (2015). Incivility as bullying in nursing education. *Nursing Science Quarterly, 28*(1), 21–26. doi:10.1177/0894318414558617 PMID:25520459

Becher, J., & Visovsky, C. (2012). Horizontal violence in nursing. *Medsurg Nursing, 21*(4), 201–232. PMID:22966523

Burger, K. G., Kramlich, D., Maltis, M., Page-Cutrara, K., & Whitfield-Harris, L. (2014). Application of the symphonological approach to faculty-to-faculty incivility in nursing education. *The Journal of Nursing Education, 53*(10), 563–568. doi:10.3928/01484834-20140922-02 PMID:25275989

Clark, C. M. (2013). National study on faculty-to-faculty incivility: Strategies to foster collegiality and civility. *Nurse Educator, 38*(3), 98–102. doi:10.1097/NNE.0b013e31828dc1b2 PMID:23608907

Cortina, L. M., Magley, V. J., Williams, J. H., & Langhout, R. D. (2001). Incivility in the workplace: Incidence and impact. *Journal of Occupational Health Psychology, 6*(1), 64–80. doi:10.1037/1076-8998.6.1.64 PMID:11199258

Del Prato, D. (2013). Students' voices: The lived experience of facility incivility as a barrier to Professional formation in associate degree nursing education. *Nurse Education Today, 33*(3), 286–290. doi:10.1016/j.nedt.2012.05.030 PMID:22726346

Dzurec, L. C., Kennison, M., & Albataineh, R. (2014). Unacknowledged threats proffered "in a manner of speaking:" Recognizing workplace bullying as shaming. *Journal of Nursing Scholarship, 46*(4), 281–291. doi:10.1111/jnu.12080 PMID:24754642

Emergency Nurses Association and Institute for Emergency Nursing Research. (2011, November). *Emergency Department Surveillance Study*. Retrieved from http://www.ncdsv.org/images/ENA_EmergencyDeptViolenceSurveillanceStudy_11-2011. pdf

Garland, D. E. (2018). The tall poppy syndrome in Orthopedics: A case report. *EC Orthopaedics, 9*(6), 376–379.

Glasper, A. (2018). Protecting healthcare staff from abuse: Tackling workplace incivility in nursing. *British Journal of Nursing (Mark Allen Publishing), 27*(22), 1336–1337. doi:10.12968/bjon.2018.27.22.1336 PMID:30525965

Green, C. (2018a). New nursing faculty and incivility: Applying mindfulness-based Strategies. *Holistic Nursing Practice, 32*(1), 4-7. doi: .0000000000000246 doi:10.1097/HNP

Green, C. (2018b). Understanding the complexities of the effects of incivility on the victim and using mindfulness to heal. *Journal of Health, Wellness, and Society*. doi:10.18848/2156-8960/CGP/v08i01/33-40

Heinrich, K. T. (2007a). Full circle moment: Recognizing the joy stealer within. *Reflections on Nursing Leadership*. Retrieved from http://www.nursingsociety.org

Heinrich, K. T. (2007b). Joy stealing: 10 mean games faculty play and how to stop the gaming. *Nurse Educator*, *32*(1), 34–38. doi:10.1097/00006223-200701000-00010 PMID:17220766

Institute of Medicine. (2003). *Keeping patients safe: Transforming the work environment for nurses*. Washington, DC: The National Academies Press.

Koharchik, L. (2018). Nursing instructor incivility toward students. *The American Journal of Nursing*, *118*(7), 64–66. doi:10.1097/01.NAJ.0000541442.76122.e4 PMID:29957646

Lachman, V. D. (2008). Whistleblowers: Troublemakers or virtuous nurses? *Dermatology Nursing*, *20*(5), 394–396. PMID:19051787

Lachman, V. D. (2014). Ethical Issues in the Disruptive Behaviors of Incivility, Bullying, and Horizontal/Lateral Violence. *Medsurg Nursing*, *23*(1), 56–60. PMID:24707670

LaSala, K. B., Wilson, V., & Sprunk, E. (2016). Nursing Academic Administrators' Lived Experiences With Incivility and Bullying From Faculty. *Nurse Educator*, *41*(3), 120–124. doi:10.1097/NNE.0000000000000234 PMID:26673315

Luparell, S. (2011). Incivility in nursing: The connection between academia and clinical settings. *American Association of Critical Care Nurses*, *31*(2), 92–95. doi:10.4037/ccn2011171 PMID:21459868

Mancl, A. C., & Pennington, B. (2011). Tall poppies in the workplace: Communication strategies used by envious others in response to successful women. *Qualitative Research Reports in Communication*, *12*(1), 79–86. do i:10.1080/17459435.2011.601701

Meires, J. (2018a). Workplace incivility: When students bully faculty. *Urologic Nursing*, *35*(5), 251–255. doi:10.7257/1053-816X.2018.38.5.251

Meires, J. (2018b). The essentials: Nursing faculty who bully students and colleagues. *Urologic Nursing*, *38*(6), 303–306. doi:10.7257/1053-816X.2018.38.6.303

Nursing Solutions, Incorporated. (2016). *National healthcare retention and RN staffing report*. Accessed June 6, 2017 http://www.nsinursingsolutions.com/Files/assets/library/retention-institute/NationalHealthcareRNRetentionReport2016.pdf

Occupational Safety and Health Administration. (2015). *Workplace violence in health care: Understanding the challenge*. Retrieved from https://www.osha.gov/Publications/OSHA3826.pdf

Palos, G. (2012). Stopping the Culture of Workplace Incivility in Nursing. *Clinical Journal of Oncology Nursing*, *16*(6), 638–639. doi:10.1188/12.CJON.638-639 PMID:23178358

Peters, A. B. (2014). Faculty to Faculty incivility: Experiences of novice nurse faculty in academia. *Journal of Professional Nursing*, *30*(3), 213–227. doi:10.1016/j.profnurs.2013.09.007 PMID:24939331

Rainford, W.C., Wood, S., McMullen, P.C., & Philipsen, N.D. (n.d.). The disruptive force of lateral violence in the health care setting. *Journal of Nursing Practice, 11*(2), 157–164.

Rodwell, J., & Demir, D. (2012). Psychological consequences of bullying for hospital and aged- care nurses. *International Nursing Review*, *59*(4), 539–546. doi:10.1111/j.1466-7657.2012.01018.x PMID:23134139

Sauer, P. A., & McCoy, T. P. (2018). Nurse bullying and intent to leave. *Nursing Economics*, *36*(5), 219–224.

The Joint Commission. (2008). Behaviors that undermine a culture of safety. *Sentinel Event Alert, 40*, 1-3. Retrieved from https://www.jointcommission.org/assets/1/18/SEA_40.PDF

The Joint Commission. (2012). *Improving patient and worker safety: Opportunities for synergy, collaboration, and innovation*. Retrieved from https://www.jointcommission.org/assets/1/18/TJC-ImprovingPatientAndWorkerSafety-Monograph.pdf

The Joint Commission. (2018). *About The Joint Commission*. Retrieved from https://www.jointcommission.org/about_us/about_the_joint_commission_main.aspx

Thomas, C. A. (2018). Stifled learning: Nursing students' experience of incivility in clinical education. *Journal of Christian Nursing*, *35*(2), 106–111. doi:10.1097/CNJ.0000000000000477 PMID:29521907

Wieland, D., & Beitz, J. M. (2015). Resilience to Social Bullying in Academia: A phenomenological Study. *Nurse Educator*, *40*(6), 289–293. doi:10.1097/NNE.0000000000000169 PMID:25950796

Wilson, B. L., Diedrich, A., Phelps, C. L., & Choi, M. (2011). Bullies at Work. *The Journal of Nursing Administration*, *41*(11), 453–458. doi:10.1097/NNA.0b013e3182346e90 PMID:22033314

Workplace Bullying Institute. (2014). *2014 WBI U.S. Workplace Bullying Survey February 2014*. Retrieved from http://www.workplacebullying.org/wbiresearch/wbi-2014-us-survey/

Wright, M., & Hill, L. H. (2014). Academic Incivility Among Health Sciences Faculty. *Adult Learning*, 14–20. doi:10.1177/1045159514558410

APPENDIX 1

Figure 1. Melting anguish

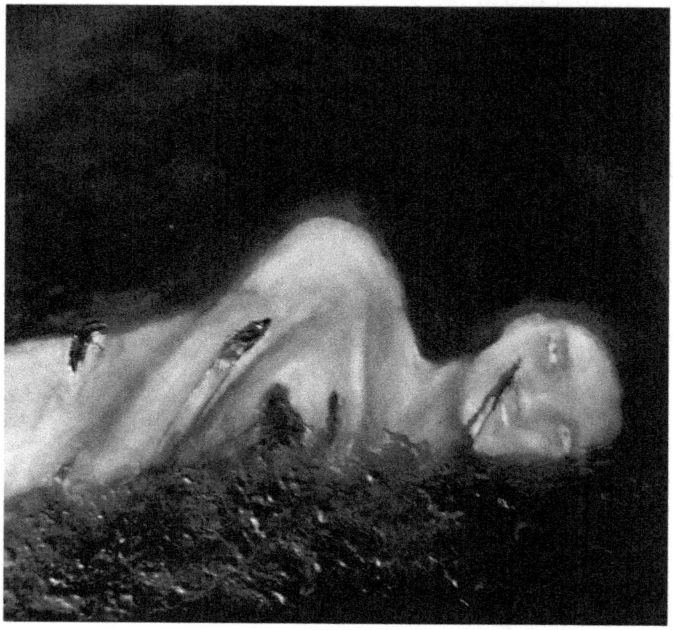

APPENDIX 2

Exploration Activities

Directions: The purpose of the *Exploration Activities* are to encourage reflection on the issue of uncivil conduct in nursing by recording one's feelings about the act of incivility.

Where do you work?

What is your role at your job? (i.e. Charge Nurse, Supervisor, Bedside Nurse, Administrator, Manager)

____

____

How has incivility impacted your work life?

____

____

____

____

____

____

How has incivility impacted your personal life?

____

____

____

____

____

____

____

If you are a nurse working directly with patients, has your experience with being bullied in the workplace impacted your ability to provide quality and safe care to patients?

____

____

____

____

____

____

____

Are you ever anxious or nervous to attend meetings or go to work when you know that you will be in contact with the person(s) bullying you?

Have you ever observed someone being treated disrespectfully in the workplace?

If you have observed a co-worker or other person being mistreated within the workplace, how did this make you feel?

What was your response to having observed someone being treated disrespectfully in the workplace? Did you notify a supervisor or someone in an administrative position?

If you made the conscious decision not to intervene, why did you make this decision?

Prior to reading this chapter, were you aware that organizations like the American Nurses Association, The Joint Commission, the Workplace Bullying Institute, Institute of Medicine, and Occupational Safety and Health Administration are against workplace bullying and support cultures of safety for workers and patients? If you were not, how does your now having this knowledge, impact your response to workplace incivility?

As a nurse, did you realize that uncivil conduct in the workplace is not supported by the American Nurses Association within the professional code of ethics?

Have you ever had a patient(s) not have a positive outcome or their length of inpatient hospitalization be increased because of a preventable medical error that likely occurred secondary to incivility in the health care environment?

How can you make a difference in changing the culture of bullying in your workplace?

If you are new faculty within academia, have you experienced bullying from your assigned mentor or other senior faculty? Or, do you feel supported?

____

____

____

Consider how your transition from clinical practice is proceeding. If you are having difficulty coping, are frequently ill and have a poor work-life balance, consider talking to someone. Do not remain alone in your struggle or isolate. There are likely other faculty that have experienced the same struggles that you are going through. Coping strategies will be discussed in other chapters.

Student nurses can experience incivility in nursing school from peers, faculty, and on the clinical unit from nursing staff and other disciplines. Have you experienced incivility within any of these settings?

____

____

____

As a student nurse, if you have experienced incivility, have you spoken to anyone about how these negative interactions have made you feel?

____

____

____

The rigor of nursing school can be emotionally and physically demanding. If you are experiencing bullying, it is important to use the Counseling Services available on campus and discuss in a safe place, the issues you are dealing with and with whom. Also, go to your campus Student Affairs Office and the Coordinator or Chair of your nursing program to discuss concerns as well. Please know that you are not alone.

Chapter 3
Health and Mental Health

ABSTRACT

As healthcare organizations use approaches such as structural empowerment theory and nurse residency programs to engage new graduate nurses in becoming productive members of the organizational culture, bullying and incivility experienced by these nurses can undermine organizations' efforts. Chapter 3 introduces the Reporting of Uncivil Conduct Chain of Command to provide support and direction to nurses that are experiencing bullying by perpetrators in the workplace. Unresolved and persistent uncivil conduct can result in health and mental health problems for affected nurses. Hence, in order to protect nurses' overall health and safety, it is necessary for organizations to adopt zero tolerance for bullying and incivility. Additionally, nurses may benefit from screening programs that can identify risks for self-harm secondary to stress and depression that could be caused by incivility in the workplace.

INTRODUCTION

Incivility impacts the health and mental health of affected nurses. For nurses, increased call-outs from work because of fatigue, frustration, anxiety, and depression associated with being bullied, not only places constraints on their colleagues, but impacts patient care. Annually, healthcare organizations have a financial loss of as much as $30,000 to $100,000 (Becher & Visovsky 2012) for each employee that has been effected by incivility within the workplace.

The very nature of the nursing profession and the interactions that nurses daily have with patients, families, and other health disciplines, can be

DOI: 10.4018/978-1-5225-7341-8.ch003

emotionally and physically demanding. Nurses must arrive at the workplace attentive, well rested, and physically capable to complete patient assessments (i.e. physical, neurological, withdrawal from substances or alcohol), perform skilled care (i.e. wound dressings, administration of intravenous medications), and meet the psychosocial needs of patients and their family members. Bullying distracts nurses from performing well, the job they were trained to do, providing health care to patients.

Uncivil Behaviors Psychological Impact

Oyeleye, Hanson, O'Connor, and Dunn (2013) conducted a quantitative study using exploratory correlational methods. The purpose of the study was to explore the relationship of stress, burnout, and workplace incivility on nurses' turnover intentions (decision to leave their job) and psychological empowerment. A total of 61 nurses participated in the study; 87% (n= 53) were female and 28% (n= 8) were male. The ages of the participants ranged from 23 to 61 years and participants' races were white (n= 50, 82%), other, (n=1, 2%), African American (n=3, 5%), and Asian (n= 7, 12%). The nurses' years of experience in the profession varied from 1 year to 40 years.

Oyeleye et al. (2013) used the following five instruments in the study: Maslach Burnout Inventory (MBI), the Uncivil Workplace Incivility Scale (WIS), Spreitzer Psychological Empowerment Scale (PES), the Perceived Stress Scale (PSS10), and a Turnover Intention scale. Results indicated that there were statistically significant correlations between stress and burnout (p= .000), burnout and turnover intention (p= .005), and stress and incivility (p=.001). Study findings suggest that nurses experiencing increases in burnout and stress may leave their jobs.

Kang, Jeong, and Kong (2018) conducted a qualitative study using a grounded theory approach (Corbin and Strauss, 2015) to explore nursing students' experiences with incivility. Sixteen nursing students participated. The 16 nursing students had all experienced incivility during their clinical placement. Kang et al. (2018) invited the students to participate in one-on-one interviews. Results indicated that nursing students felt they were outsiders within the organizational hierarchy and culture of their clinical placement. Students verbalized feeling marginalized and in response became passive, submissive, and shocked that incivility had occurred in a professional setting.

Kang et al. (2018) concluded that when nursing students experience incivility during their academic preparation to enter the profession of nursing, their identity is threatened. Students undergo role conflict and have low self-esteem. Study findings suggest that nursing students that experience incivility should be provided counseling services and educational programs be developed by nursing programs to address the incivility and offer coping strategies. Schools of nursing are recommended to have guidelines that ensure students learn within supportive clinical environments that they feel safe within.

Structural Empowerment

Structural empowerment is a theory that views workplaces that empower employees as having a positive impact on work performance (Kanter, 1977). Power in the workplace can be attained both through informal and formal ways. Employees exhibit informal power when they form interpersonal allegiances and networks of peer groups, with subordinates and superiors within their organization, as well as outside of the organization. Formal power occurs within an organization when employees have roles that are visible and align with organizational missions and vision statements, and employees have jobs that have flexibility. According to Kanter (1977), employees tend to thrive, have job satisfaction, and are committed to their organizations success, when opportunities to learn and grow professionally are made available to them.

Structural empowerment, although developed in 1977, has been referenced within new graduate nurse residency programs such as the American Association of Colleges of Nursing Vizient (2019) programs, in the development of evidenced-based practice (EBP) projects as a prerequisite for completion of residency programs. The length of residency programs are usually one year and culminate in EBP projects such as unit-based reduction of central access device infections or examining ways to reduce turnover intentions. These EBP projects are presented to the new graduate nurses' colleagues and key stakeholders within the organization (i.e. Vice President of Nursing Services, Chief Nursing Officers, Nurse Managers, or Healthcare Providers). Structural empowerment can be instrumental in health care facilities retaining nurses through engagement with their units and the organization as a whole.

Wing, Regan, and Laschinger (2015), used a predictive, non-experimental design to examine structural empowerment in relation to workplace incivility and new graduate nurses experience of mental health symptoms. Their sample size was 394 new graduate nurses working within a hospital in Ontario, Canada. Instruments used were the following: the Conditions for Work Effectiveness Questionnaire (CWEQ-II, Laschinger et al., 2001) to measure structural empowerment, the Workplace Incivility Scale (WIS, Cortina et al., 2001), and the State of Mind subscale from the Pressure Manager Indicator (PMI, Williams & Cooper, 1998). The CWEQ measured structural empowerment and had Cronbach alphas that range between 0.78 to 0.94. The WIS assessed incivility that was experienced by the new graduate nurses in their interactions with co-workers and supervisors. And lastly, PMI measured anxiety and depressive symptoms experienced by the new graduate nurses.

Wing et al. (2015) found that high levels of structural empowerment experienced by new graduate nurses, was associated with less mental health symptoms. Incivility experienced by the new graduate nurses, by supervisors and co-workers, was found to diminish the positive effect of the work environment. Hence, although health care facilities can strategically set in place, positive opportunities (i.e. training, promotions, awards, and career ladders) for nurses to grow and learn, uncivil behaviors in the workplace still can negatively impact the mental health of new graduate nurses.

An Attack on One's Self-Concept

Perpetrators of incivility seek to discredit their targets professionally by openly questioning their expertise (public humiliation) and knowledge in front of others. Additionally, the perpetrator may seek to sabotage the completion of work in progress or take credit (destabilization) for the nurse(s) work for whom they are bullying (TJC, 2016; WBI, 2016). Perpetrators further isolate their targets by withholding information. The latter behaviors can cause nurses that are experiencing bullying in the workplace to feel physically ill and mentally fatigued, anxious and depressed.

Case Study 4 is a hypothetical case study on workplace incivility. All characters within the case study are fictional. This case study explores the transition of a new graduate nurse from the academic environment to clinical practice.

Case Study 4: Maria

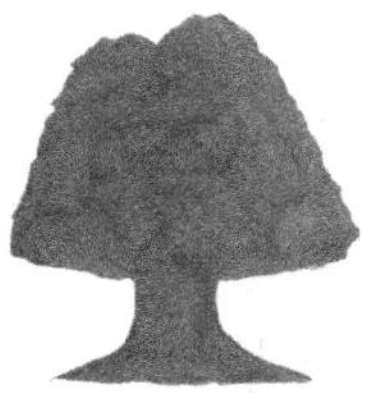

Maria graduated from college with a bachelor of science in nursing 11 months ago. She was hired to work at a large teaching hospital within her desired specialization of critical care nursing. Maria relocated from a small town in the south, to a large metropolitan city in the north of the United States. Maria's orientation to her unit was comprehensive and her preceptor Ann was a critical care nurse for 31 years and enjoyed teaching her.

Maria's preceptor Ann was supportive, engaging, and provided her with opportunities to learn new skills daily. Ann and Maria even attended critical care conferences together. Maria had learned so much quickly, that her patients would inquire how long she had been a nurse because she was so confident and knowledgeable.

Ann, after commending Maria on her progression after 10 months of preceptorship, informed Maria that she would be retiring. After Ann retired, Maria still felt confident and enjoyed coming to work each day. One day, as Maria was talking to a patient and their family member, another nurse entered the patient's hospital room and started correcting the information that Maria had just provided. Maria felt humiliated and quickly excused herself and exited the room.

When Maria later approached the nurse to ask why she had interrupted her as she was talking to her patient, the nurse laughed and walked away. The nurse repeated this behavior the following week with a different patient. Although Maria tried to ignore the behaviors, the situation escalated out of control as the nurse began challenging her skills and humiliating her in front of co-workers and healthcare providers.

Maria hated going to work. She was depressed and felt alone and isolated. Maria developed acid reflux and experienced headaches. Her thoughts both at home and at work focused on the incivility she was experiencing at work.

Maria's nurse manager asked to meet with her after noticing on the unit schedule that she had begun to call-out from work ill several times during a one-month period. Maria was tearful as she explained to her manager what had happened and how the bullying she had been enduring had affected her health. The nurse manager instructed Maria to begin documenting the dates and times the bullying occurred and who was present. Three months after the bullying had begun, it abruptly ended when the nurse was placed on progressive disciplinary action by the nurse manager for uncivil conduct within the workplace.

The perpetrating nurse was placed on a different shift than Maria. The two nurses did not interact. Maria's acid reflux eventually resolved and her depression gradually lifted. Maria learned from this experience the importance of addressing bullying behaviors immediately. In addition, the necessity of informing a supervisor or manager of the bullying as soon as possible.

Maria' Story—Addressing the Problem

Maria's experience with being bullied in the workplace ended when a nurse manager, while addressing Maria's pattern of sick call-outs, discovered that Maria was experiencing incivility. Nurses being bullied in the workplace may feel isolated and that no one cares. This perception (Moola, Ehlers, & Hattingh, 2008) is not always accurate because it is clouded by the stress nurses experience related to the uncivil behavior from perpetrators. It is often when nurses begin to share their story of incivility experiences with a trusted source (i.e. a counselor, manager, peer, Human Resources representative), that healing can begin and recognition of the inappropriateness of the perpetrator's behavior can be processed and validated.

Nurse Residency Programs

Nurses that live in silence and tolerate the bullying, are at risk for not only physical and mental health problems, but job stress and burnout (Wu et al., 2007; Chen, Lin, Wang, & Hou, 2009). For retention of new graduate nurses, it is imperative that they receive support in addressing incivility during their period of orientation and acclamation to the nursing role. Many health care facilities, in response to the need to support new graduates and retention, have developed nurse residency programs.

The purpose of nurse residency programs are to support the Institute of Medicine (IOM, 2003) and Quality and Safety Education for Nurses (QSEN, 2019) initiatives of introducing patient-centered care, evidenced-based practice, informatics, quality improvement, safety, and teamwork and collaboration (QSEN, 2019) to new graduate nurses (and experienced nurses re-entering the field). Nurse residency programs focus on the development of nurses' roles within health care systems, evidenced-based practice, leadership skills, and awareness of how their work and roles impact patients' health outcomes. Nurse residency programs, have been instrumental in decreasing new graduate nurse turnover and preparing nurses to apply critical thinking and decision-making skills within the clinical environment (Vizient/AACN, 2016; Vizient/AACN, 2019).

Within nurse residency programs, new graduate nurses are trained in cohorts. The establishment of cohort training facilitates connectedness among the new graduates and creates a forum whereby the nurses can safely share their experiences on the clinical units; positive and negative, this includes incivility. For new graduate nurse Maria, sharing with her cohort or a member(s) of the cohort, could have also helped her address the uncivil conduct on her unit.

Coordinators of nurse residency programs are a wonderful resource for new nurses because they can maintain objectivity. The sole purpose of the coordinator role is to prepare new graduate nurses and nurses re-entering the nursing profession (or a new clinical area of practice) with their transition to the health care facility. Coordinators of nurse residency programs may hire the part-time assistance of what are referred to as nurse residency facilitators. Nurse residency facilitators are experienced nurses that meet with hired nurses to facilitate discussions on planned topics that the nurses may experience within the clinical environments such as when *patients' conditions decline, coping with the loss of a patient, providing support to family members in crisis, or coping with difficult relationships* in the health care environment.

Nurse residency programs are instrumental in helping new graduate nurses and nurses re-entering the field, recognize the importance of communication skills, respect in the workplace, coping with stress, self-care, being unafraid to challenge their colleagues when a potential procedural error is identified (i.e. a break in sterility during a surgical procedure or dressing change) or they disagree with a treatment regimen prescribed for a patient. The number of skills taught are too many to write. Nurse residency programs also encourage scholarly research, as nurse cohorts work collaboratively to identify areas in need of improvement on their units and develop EBP quality improvement projects that contribute greatly to patients and staff on their designated units they work on, as well as the health care facility itself.

Nurse residency programs serve as a reminder of the responsibility that each nurse has to educate the next generation of nurse professionals. New nurses must be well-informed of the nature of bullying in the workplace and the necessity of having an intolerance for incivility. Change begins with every nurse from multiple generations, novice to expert alike.

Case Study 5 is a hypothetical case study. All characters within this case study are fictional. This case study provides an example of a nurse who is a caregiver of older parents that must contend with bullying in the workplace.

Case Study 5: Maritza

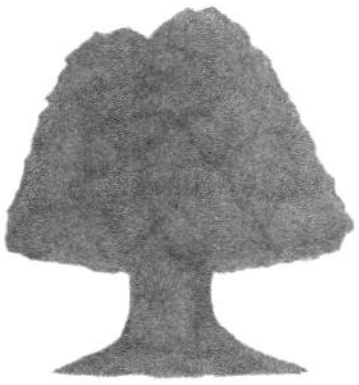

Maritza has been a nurse for 32 years. She recently relocated to Florida from North Carolina to care for her aging parents. After three months residing in Florida, her father died of a heart attack. Maritza then became the primary caretaker for her mother who has Alzheimer's disease.

Maritza worked day shift at a local hospital and hired a nurse assistant as a companion to provide care to her mother while she was at work. Her mother became combative and paranoid. The nurse assistant was assaulted by Maritza's mother on a daily basis for a week and Maritza's mother constantly accused the nurse assistant of stealing money and jewelry. One day Maritza received a phone call at work from the agency that the nurse assistant was employed, and was informed that it was unsafe for them to provide companions for her mother. Effective that day, the companion service ended.

Martiza spoke with her nurse manager and assistant nurse manager about her dilemma. It was perfect timing, an evening shift nurse had resigned so Maritza took this position and started two days later. Working in the evening allowed Maritza to provide care to her mother during the day and provide overnight care of her mother as well. A neighbor who was a retired nurse, agreed to take care of her mother while she was at work. Maritza paid her neighbor $500.00 a week.

Ann, a new graduate nurse was hired to work the evening shift. Ann was very bossy and opinionated. She had already worked in three different hospitals since graduating 18 months ago. She was not experienced enough to make the clinical decisions she attempted to make on some of the unit's complex postoperative patient cases on the surgical unit. However, Ann, a skilled liar, would falsify her level of experience and clinical competency.

Concerned that Ann's lack of integrity and ethics could eventually place a patient or patients at risk for harm, Maritza decided to go and speak with the assistant nurse manager. The assistant nurse manager and Maritza spoke at length about ways to help Ann adjust to her role on the unit and feel more comfortable seeking advice and assistance with patient care from more experienced nursing staff.

I Don't Need Your Help

The following evening, Ann approached Maritza and pushed her left shoulder from behind, startling Maritza. Ann stated, "Oops, my mistake Maritza! By the way, do me a favor, don't talk about me to my boss and no, I don't need your help." Ann then walked down the hallway quietly as if the interaction had never taken place.

One evening after work as Maritza went into the hospital parking garage to prepare to go home, she noticed a deep scratch, on the driver's side of her car that covered the full car length. The following week, her tires were slashed. Maritza reported to the hospital security what had occurred. Because of the angle of the garage camera, the perpetrator could not be identified. As a caregiver to her elderly mother, Maritza was already stressed. However, the vandalism had taken her stress to a different level, as Maritza now feared for her safety.

Maritza went to the Police Department to report the damage to her car. She was recommended to park her car in a well-lit area within the garage with clear visualization from a camera in the garage. Maritza began arriving early at work to secure parking near the surveillance cameras. Within nine days, Maritza's driver side window was smashed, glass covering the seat floor and dashboard. This time, surveillance cameras had a direct view, and a visitor exiting the garage on foot to spend the night with an ill family member had witnessed the event and reported it to a hospital security officer. Maritza was immediately notified.

Hospital security viewed the surveillance camera footage the following day and saw Ann, Maritza's co-worker, smashing her car window with a hammer. Maritza was informed, the police were contacted by the hospital security department and a statement was taken on the grounds of the hospital. The witness' description of the perpetrator and picture on camera, confirmed that it was Ann, Maritza's co-worker.

Ann was arrested and in court, denied any wrong doing. She later faced charges and Maritza acquired a restraining order. The hospital fired Ann. Maritza had no further problems, but the physical pushing and destructive damage to her car, left her shaken.

When Bullying Becomes Violent

When perpetrators physically lay hands on victims with the intention of intimidation or to do harm, it is important that these incidences are documented and reported. Maritza did not report the pushing incident on the unit, and Ann continued to escalate her attacks by damaging Maritza's property, her car. If a victim of bullying in anyway feels threatened for their safety or the safety of others in their workplace, follow the report of uncivil conduct (see Diagram 1.) chain of command and involve hospital security and or the police to document the pattern of deviant behaviors. Of concern would be if the bullying leads to self-harm or harm of others. Reported, deviant behaviors can be addressed and the perpetrators, witnesses, and victims, kept safe.

Professionalism and Confrontation

Nurses are encouraged in workplaces, to follow the chain of command. The chain of command consists of a hierarchy of leadership established for the maintenance of function and order within institutions. By following a chain of command, issues can potentially be rectified employee-to-employee, prior to being escalated to a manager, director, president, or vice president of a health care facility. Figure 1 is an example of a chain of command in an organization.

The restoration of order is the goal of the chain of command within organizations. Whenever possible, nurses should seek a solution to the bullying with the offending nurse. This provides the offending nurse the opportunity to explain their behavior, and if in fact they are aware of the implications of their patterns of communication. If bullying persists, nurses should then meet with their immediate manager or supervisor to discuss the situation.

The Hollow

Incivility may cause the affected individual to feel hurt, sad, misunderstood, and embittered. These feelings can be referred to as *the hollow*. *The hollow*, accompanied by perseveration of incidences of negative behaviors from

Figure 1. Reporting uncivil conduct chain of command

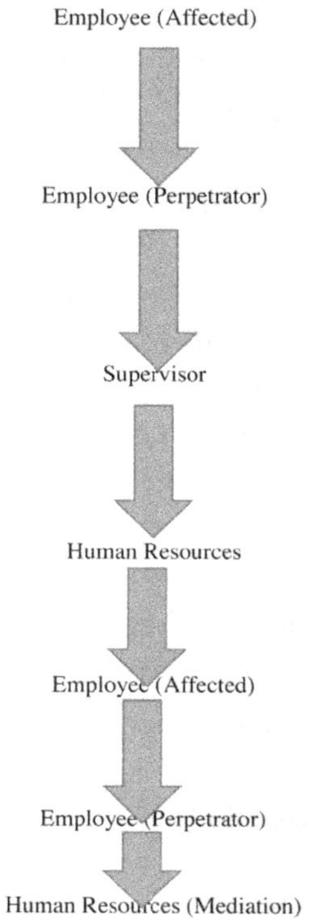

the perpetrator to the victimized nurse, can lead to illness; both mental and physical. For nurses experiencing *the hollow*, symptomatically, they tend to lack energy, enthusiasm, and focus. These symptoms arise in-part, because of the perseveration component of the hollow. As nurses mentally recall negative words said to them and the situations in which they felt vulnerable and attacked by the bullying perpetrator, anxiety and frustration are heighted, as events are replayed over and over again.

The Hollow and Work Productivity

The term *the hollow* was created by the author to explain symptomatology that victims of incivility can experience. Nurses may feel overwhelmed by the bully's continuous attacks on their character and their abilities to perform the job. This can lead to nurses having the sensation that they are sinking and enveloped in deep sadness. Nurses affected by *the hollow* may experience intermittent periods of worry and anxiety, accompanied by perseveration on events at work involving the bully or bullies, and intermittent tearfulness.

Nurses experiencing *the hollow* will inevitably, have a change in their work productivity. Preoccupied in their thoughts with perseveration of the incidences of negative bullying interactions, affected nurses may have a decrease in their ability to concentrate, think logically, and think analytically. The danger of *the hollow* for nurses that are in direct care practice, is that intellectually, nurses' thought processes may become clouded and they may have difficulty critically thinking within the clinical environment. The latter may compromise nurses care of patients related to their disrupted thought processes, secondary to *the hollow*.

Nurses can overcome the feelings associated with *the hollow* by either deciding to leave their work environment shared with the perpetrator(s), request a change of shifts to avoid all interaction with the perpetrator(s), or report the perpetrator(s) and seek the mediation help of a nurse manager or Human Resource Department representative. Additionally, nurses should seek counseling through their company's employee assistance programs (EAP). Untreated, *the hollow* can develop into a clinical depression.

Case Study 6 is a hypothetical case study and all characters are fictional. In this case study, Alice, a nurse employed within a surgical intensive care unit (SICU) experiences bullying by her mentor and other nurses on the unit. Alice must learn self-care as she endures the bullying and incivility.

Case Study 6: Alice

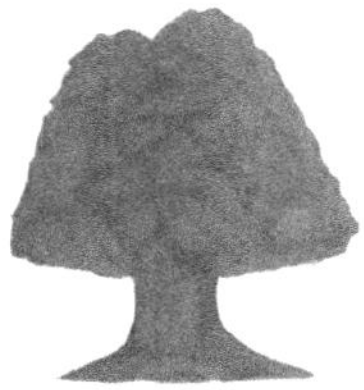

Alice experienced bullying on her job. The bullying started shortly after she was hired to work as a critical care nurse within a surgical intensive care unit (SICU). Alice's bullies were four nurses; one of the four was her mentor. The nurses would go out of their way to attempt to prove that Alice was incompetent in front of not only her patients and other healthcare disciplines, but other nursing colleagues. Alice had never did anything to these women. She did not have work a history with them or anyone in the hospital for that matter. Alice was new to the state and institution after deciding to relocate one year ago after a divorce.

For Alice, relocating to a new state seemed exciting since her ex-husband and she had no children; this was truly like starting over. Alice had worked as a critical care nurse for 10 years before marrying her former husband. She was an experienced nurse who was certified within her specialization.

Alice was already emotionally fragile when she relocated secondary to the divorce, so the bullying made it even more difficult. One evening as Alice prepared to leave work after completing a 12-hour shift, she walked into the nurses' breakroom to get a cup of coffee. She did not see that one of the perpetrators had placed their foot in the way to trip her. Alice fell and hot coffee spilled all over the floor and onto her uniform.

Alice informed her nurse manager about the bullying and that it was escalating, but her complaints seemingly were ignored. The perpetrators were comfortable bullying others because it was tolerated on the unit. No one questioned the perpetrators' behaviors.

Alice went to speak to Human Resources (HR) about the problem and they instructed her to "keep track of the incidences." Alice documented the dates and times of incidences and if a witness was present. The HR representative suggested Alice meet again with her nurse manager to discuss the problem. Alice met with the nurse manager who listened to her concerns, but did nothing.

Alice was not sleeping well, had lost weight, and had difficulty concentrating. She had a few friends in the apartment building she lived within and had shared with one, a nurse that worked at another hospital, what was happening at work. Alice's friend recommended she contact an attorney. Alice did not contact an attorney and continued to reach out to HR, but to no avail. Alice applied for a position on the cardiac intensive care unit (CCU); however, Alice's nurse manager delayed the transfer to the CCU because the SICU had a shortage of staff.

Alice seldom felt happy and was anxious upon arriving at work. Alice was very cautious when administering medications and completing procedures for her patients because her mind was so preoccupied with rewinding and playing back things that were said to her by the perpetrators. Alice's self-esteem and self-confidence had suffered a great deal. It was as if she had no experience in nursing at all. She felt depleted of energy and lived in a constant state of fatigue. Because Alice was alone in a new state, she felt that she could not just leave her job given her financial responsibilities.

Alice's thoughts were always racing and replaying the painful bullying events. She began to withdraw from friends, went only to work, and came home. Alice's sleep and appetite were poor. One night, while driving over a small bridge in the middle of the night coming from the grocery store,

Alice stopped her car and stood on the bridge looking at the river below. Contemplating suicide and in turmoil, she changed her mind as she thought of her parents and her Catholic faith. She decided to return to her car and proceeded home.

One day while at work, Alice went to administer a morning injection of subcutaneous heparin (Porcine) to a patient. The patient's family member informed her that the night nurse had administered the injection at 6:00 a.m. The patient was nonverbal and on a ventilator and the family member, whom normally leaves at 6:30 a.m., had forgotten his reading glasses, returned to the patient's room to obtain them. The nurse had not signed off the order, and informed Alice during handoff report at 7:05 a.m. that the 6:00 a.m. heparin injection had not been administered. Alice agreed to do the injection.

Alice asked the nurse why she had not been informed that the nurse had decided to administer the heparin injection. However, the nurse, one of Alice's perpetrators, insisted that she had not administered the medication. The family member, overhearing their discussion, reiterated the story and verified that it had been administered. The patient's spouse said to the other nurse, "You told me when you came in my wife's room at 6:00 a.m. that you were giving her heparin. Did you tell me the truth or not?"

The nurse manager, entering the unit, overheard the conversation with the family member and Alice's co-worker at the nurses' station. The nurse manager listened intently to the family member and apologized for the "mix up." Alice felt set-up and her suspicions were confirmed when one of the nurses on the night shift shared the perpetrator had informed her that she would be administering the said patient's heparin injection at 6:00 a.m., her last medication for the night shift, as they spoke in front of the medication pyxis. Alice shared this with her nurse manager who stated, "Alice, you have been nothing but trouble since you got here. You work with good nurses that try to support you, why don't you do the same."

Alice was visibly shaken with what had just occurred. She attempted to continue to work, but after this last incident, felt unsupported, betrayed, set-up, and paranoid about protecting her license. She informed the nurses she was working with, her patients and the nurse manager, that she felt ill and would be going home to rest.

Alice went home and fell asleep crying. When she awoke at 5:00 p.m., she could not believe that had slept so long. She finally felt rested after weeks of disrupted sleep. She ordered a salad and sandwich from a local deli and ate the full meal. At about 7:00 p.m., one of Alice's friends in the apartment building came to show Alice a dress she had purchased. They laughed and spoke at length over cups of tea. At 10:00 p.m., Alice cleaned her apartment and sorted through her mail. At 12:00 midnight, she took a shower.

At 3:00 a.m., Alice left her apartment building and drove over the small bridge. She stepped out of her car and looking at the calm waters, climbed on top of the bridge and jumped into the river below. At 5:30 a.m., Alice's car was discovered. Alice's body was recovered at 8:00 a.m.

Examining Alice's Case

In examining Alice's case, one of the factors that may have led to her suicide, was her being bullied at work and feeling unsupported. However, risk factors involved in her being vulnerable were her recent divorce and resulting relocation to a new state. In a new state and still healing from her marital problems, Alice's support system of family and close friends, were no longer a part of her immediate community. Alice had become increasingly emotionally fragile because of the steady escalation of the bullying and for Alice, the final incident of her being set-up to make a potential medication error by one of her perpetrators, made her feel like she had no way out of the situation. Alice left work with the plan to harm herself.

Evidence of Alice's initial contemplation of self-harm was her stopping on the small bridge and viewing the river below. After the final incident with a perpetrator at work and an interaction with the nurse manager that brought no resolution to the situation, Alice decided to end her life. Actual evidence of Alice's decision to end her life was her sudden ability to sleep without disruption, eat and enjoy a meal, have renewed energy to clean her apartment, and spend time with a friend laughing and enjoying the moment. All of the latter had been disrupted secondary to the stress Alice experienced from the workplace bullying.

The Unspoken Observations

Alice had worked at the hospital for over a year and the bullying had begun shortly after she was hired. It is likely that other nurses observed Alice being bullied in the workplace. However, no one intervened.

Nurses and Suicide

Suicide is when a person decides to end his or her own life. Rates of suicide vary considerably with regard to ethnicity, age, religion, countries in which persons reside, and sex. In 2015, suicide deaths worldwide were 1.4%, and suicide was determined to be the seventeenth cause of death (WHO, 2018). For persons aged 15 to 29 years of age, suicide is the second leading cause of death globally. Approximately 800,000 people die each year related to suicide. The World Health Organization (2018), in examination of indicators for adult suicide, noted that for every successful suicide, there are about 20 self-harm attempts.

Rates and frequency of suicide were trended by occupation. The determination of rates of suicide were calculated by age and sex. According to McIntosh et al. (2016), persons working in the fishing industries, forestry, and farming were at the highest risk for suicide. The overall suicide rate for this group was 84.5 per 100,000 population and 90.5 males. For females, protective service occupations had the highest risk for suicide at 14.1. Library, training, and education had the lowest rates of suicide at 7.5.

A United Kingdom study performed in England over a period of five years; 2011 to 2015, examined occupation, gender, and age in relation to suicide. Results indicated that males within health professions, had a lower risk of suicide (16% lower risk, with a 37% lowered risk for males that were identified as medical practitioners). However, females in health professions risk for suicide was 24% higher than the female national average. The occupation of nursing was the reason the suicide risks was 23% higher than the national average; female health professionals often chose poisoning as a means to end their lives (Windsor-Shellard, 2017).

A National Academy of Medicine (NAM) discussion paper written by Davidson, Mendis, Stuck, DeMichele, and Zisook (2018), examined the lack of information available in the literature on suicides within the nursing profession. The authors conducted an internet search on suicide by rates, year and occupation within the United States. Data examined occupations that provided services to the public. These are the following professions that data were found on during the internet search: military officer (combat infantry closed to women- 37.2/100,000; combat infantry, engineer never deployed and closed to women- 41.2/100,000; combat support medical- 18.5/100,000, all data from 2004-2009), police officer (108 per year, 2016), physician (300 to 400 per year, data from 2015 to 2016), and educator (63 per year, data from 2011). No data were found on nurses.

There are approximately 3.4 million practicing nurses within the United States (ANA, 2017). Statistically, hospitals tend to trend data regarding nurses such as, injuries sustained on the job (worker's compensation), turnover in the hiring of nurses, and stress and burnout risks within the profession of nursing. However, when a nurse self-injures and ultimately commits suicide, none of these data are available by health care facilities. According to Davidson et al. (2018), for nurses that commit suicide, whispers of their death are heard among colleagues and no data to interpret the potential meaning of their loss of life, is known.

Nursing is a profession of caring whereby relationships are developed daily among colleagues, patients' families, and patients. The nurse regularly interfaces between varieties of different disciplines. Nurses must daily meet the needs of patients and the expectations of healthcare systems, while coping with deaths of patients and peers they have grown close to. Nurses may also be attempting to thrive in work situations where they have had to cope with the criticism of other nurses, resulting in low self-esteem and disempowerment.

Suicide risks for nurses are similar to those of the public (CDC, 2018). For example, nurses that have a mental (or physical) illness may be at risk for self-harm during periods of exacerbation of symptoms and stress. Also, if a nurse has a history of addiction to drugs or alcohol, these also put the nurse at risk for poor impulse control and self-harm. Nurses that have a history of a relative that successfully committed suicide are also at risk for self-harm as well. Of greater concern for nurses that are suicidal is their clinical knowledge, skills, and accessibility to lethal means to end their lives. For example, nurses have access to a variety of different drugs via pills, injections, sublingual, transdermal patches, and intravenous routes that can abruptly end one's life.

Because of the daily physical, emotional, and spiritual intensity of the nursing profession, nurses experiencing personal problems at home such as divorce, caring for an ill family member, or child-rearing issues, may feel overwhelmed. As the nurse begins to feel overwhelmed, hopelessness and helplessness may become central to their daily thought processes, leaving the nurse feeling depressed. It is when the nurse feels depressed, hopeless and helpless, the potential contemplation for a plan of suicide (suicidal ideation), may develop.

Nurses can be educated on how to recognize and help other nurses who may be at risk for self-harm. Becoming aware of potential warning signs for suicide is a proactive way of understanding how to intervene to keep nurses alive. The following are examples of warning signs:

1. The nurse is preoccupied with dying and death; discussing people who have died or perhaps examining websites or YouTube videos about death
2. The nurse no longer takes an interest in their appearance and may even appear disheveled at times
3. The nurse begins to take risks that are unwarranted such as jumping off a cliff to swim or bungee jumping
4. The nurse talks about having difficulty sleeping and a change in appetite
5. The nurse has mood lability or changes in their behavior that is atypical to how they usually behave
6. The nurse no longer has an interest in work, hobbies, spending time with friends socially, or if a student, disinterested in school
7. The nurse has a prior history of a self-harm attempt
8. The nurse has recently had several losses such as the death of a spouse, child, close friend, the end of an intimate relationship with a partner, or a divorce
9. The nurse has recently suffered significant material, property, or financial loss
10. The nurse begins to use drugs and alcohol by their report, to calm themselves, for sleep and/or to reduce their stress
11. The nurse begins to give away material items of great significance to them
12. The nurse occasionally talks about suicide or brings up self-harm out of the context of a conversation focused on a different topic
13. The nurse visits a funeral home to make arrangements for death or makes out a will
14. The nurse, who is normally very religious, stops going to church and reading their primary religious text (i.e. Torah, Bible, Quran)

Verbalized Feelings of Suicide

Persons that are suicidal may sometimes voice their feelings, it is however important that someone listens. The subtle words of a person struggling with the decision to live or die can be misinterpreted or misunderstood. Below are statements that can be associated with a person contemplating life or death:

1. "I just can't sleep or eat anymore."
2. "This sadness just will not go away."
3. "No one pays attention to me anyway."
4. "No one listens to what I say."
5. "I just can't get my life together. It all feels out of control."
6. "I feel like I am always going to have pain in my life."
7. "I feel like no one cares for me or cares to be around me."
8. "Why would anyone think I'm smart?"
9. "I have felt depressed for a long time."
10. "It all seems so hopeless."
11. "I just feel so ambivalent about everything. I don't know how I am going to make this decision."
12. "I just cannot gather my thoughts."
13. "I am just in so much emotional and physical pain."
14. "I don't think there are any solutions. I just need to be left alone."
15. "This bullying has become too much for me to deal with. I feel like no one is ever going to help me."

Nurses Supporting Nurses

The American Nurses Association's Code of Ethics encourages collegiality among nurses. For nurses identifying and supporting colleagues at risk for self-harm, it is important to help affected nurses get help. Nurses experiencing the stress of bullying in addition to the normal stress of their job as a nurse and personal life stressors, may feel hopeless. Below are interventions that nurses can implement in helping other nurses who are contemplating suicide:

1. Discuss with the nurse that there are other alternatives
2. Immediately remove stockpiled pills, knives, guns, or other items that can be used by the nurse to harm themselves
3. Never promise to break a confidence or be sworn to secrecy
4. Never dare the nurse to harm themselves
5. Make yourself available for support
6. Show an interest in the nurse's health and well-being
7. Obtain assistance from agencies or a professional that has a specialization in suicide prevention and crisis intervention
8. Never come off as being judgmental toward your nurse colleague
9. Listen intently as they express their feelings. Do not judge them or offer your opinion

10. Openly discuss suicide and suicidal ideation. Ask your nurse colleague directly whether they are having thoughts of self-harm
11. Ask your nurse colleague if they have a plan to harm themselves. If they answer yes, ask them to describe the plan
12. Never act surprised or shocked about the nurse's disclosure of, or attempt to self-harm. Keep the conversation(s) open

Getting the Suicidal Nurse Help

When exploring available services for nurses who are at risk for self-harm, it is important to be aware of crisis intervention and available professionals in the surrounding area that are convenient and easily accessible. There are crisis intervention services available in every state. For nurses, it may be helpful to begin with contacting a professional through their employer's employment assistance program (EAP). For nurses that do not desire any contact directly or indirectly related to their employment, the Federal Communications Commission (2017) offers the dialing of 2-1-1, as a means to obtain information on available human service agencies in their local area. The 2-1-1 number is accessible to over 270 million people within the United States, Puerto Rico, and the District of Columbia. For nurses unaware if 211 is available in their local area, go to the 211 website, www.211.org.

The National Suicide Prevention Lifeline (NSPL, 2018) is a 24 hour service offered seven days a week. The NSPL is available to provide emotional support to persons in crisis. All information is confidential. The NSPL also provides information on available services within person's immediate areas where they reside, for crisis intervention. For nurses assisting nurses that may be struggling with thoughts of suicide, the NSPL number is 1-800-273-Talk.

Nurse Workplace Bullying and Incivility and the HEAR Program

In exploring a potential program that can be used to assist nurses that may be at risk for self-harm secondary to workplace bullying and incivility, the Healer Education, Assessment and Referral (HEAR) program can be an option. The HEAR program is used to identify doctors that are at risk for self-harm by applying two approaches in helping physicians not harm themselves. The first approach uses educational presentations on the topics of depression, suicide, and burnout. The second provides an anonymous confidential web-based assessment and screening tool for physicians to take privately. The web-based assessment and screening tool is encrypted and is an Interactive Survey Program (ISP) developed specifically to identify physicians at risk for self-harm and depression (Davidson et al., 2018).

At the University of California San Diego Health, a university affiliated health care institution, before the year 2009, each year, a faculty member, medical student, or resident, committed suicide (Davidson et al., 2018). A survey to assess the well-being of physicians was developed and findings revealed significant drinking among faculty and residents at 6%, self-reported depression at 29%, and active suicidal ideation at the rate of 3% or higher (Reinhardt, Chavez, Jackson, & Mathews, 2005). A committee was developed to investigate the creation of a program that could help prevent suicide within this population. The committee, entitled the Physician Well-being Committee (PWBC), working closely with the American Foundation for Suicide Prevention (AFSP), and developed the HEAR program (formerly known as the Suicide Prevention and Depression Awareness Program).

The HEAR program currently has helped to decrease the suicides at the University of California San Diego Health, from 1 suicide a year, to 1 suicide in 6 years. During the years 2009 to 2016, 502 medical faculty, 341 fellows, 90 residents, and 519 medical students, have completed the web-based survey. Approximately 63 met with a program counselor in person, 112 communicated online with a counselor online, and 9 spoke to a counselor on the telephone (Davidson, et al., 2018). The HEAR program is currently offered within 8 medical schools, over 60 medical teaching campuses, and continues to grow (Davidson, et al., 2018). The HEAR takes a proactive stance on suicide prevention.

Nurses, like physicians, work long hours, and have difficulty balancing their work and personal lives. Compassion fatigue, stress and burnout, workload demands, and one's own values and ethics conflicting with those of the health care organization, can also contribute to nurses feeling frustrated and depressed. Although nursing is a profession that requires collaboration with other health care disciplines and fellow nurse colleagues, nurses can feel isolated in their roles as healthcare professionals, especially when working within dysfunctional workplace cultures with bullying and lateral violence present.

Both nurses and physicians must have a keen eye for assessment and the ability to differentiate disease processes presenting in their patients with subtle symptomatology. Davidson et al. (2018) notes that persons who decide to become nurses, may have the characteristics of perfectionism and are compulsive with an acute attention to detail. While these traits can be beneficial, specifically to patients whom have placed their lives in the capable hands of these health professionals, these same traits increase the likelihood for stress.

Davidson et al. (2018) trialed the HEAR program with a participant group of nurses. Out of 2,475 nurses, 172 completed questionnaires. Upon completion of the questionnaires, data indicated that 98 (55%) nurses were at moderate risk for self-harm, 19 (11%) reported having previously attempted to harm themselves, and 12 (7%) had active thoughts or made actions to self-harm. Seventeen of these nurses agreed to receive help via a referral, for mental health treatment and 44 (26%) received either verbal or in-person counseling services. Based upon the data, nurses were found to have benefited from the HEAR program, and proactive screening for suicide is an effective means of identifying nurses at risk for self-harm.

RECOMMENDATIONS

Given the successful trial of the HEAR program with nurses, it may be beneficial for hospitals and other healthcare facilities to consider adopting this program for both nurses and physicians to promote healthy work environments. This program can help prevent self-harm with these vulnerable health professions. The HEAR program may help screen nurses whom are victims of workplace bullying. Because nurses experiencing bullying and incivility can have depression, stress, and anxiety, in addition to physiological symptoms, use of HEAR program within health care institutions may help identify these nurses early. By identifying nurses at risk for self-harm related to workplace incivility and bullying, nurses can be provided emotional support before suicide becomes an irreversible option.

Putting Yourself First

It is important that nurses put themselves first when it comes to coping and healing from experiences of bullying. Nurses who decide to place all of their energies into work solely, may feel emotionally empty and have difficulty managing frustrations related to their own victimization. For nurses experiencing uncivil conduct within the work environment, the ability to distance from the actual workplace and focus on the completion of work during actual work hours, can be healthy. Setting boundaries around self-care and the protection of one's mental and physical health, can be beneficial for affected nurses in the preservation of physiological and psychological homeostasis.

Appendix 2 contains activities that further explore job-related stress in relation to workplace bullying. Self-care and the importance of nurses being aware of suicide risks and prevention are discussed. Suicide resource support for nurses and their affected colleagues, are also provided.

REFERENCES

American Association of Colleges of Nursing. (2016). *Vizient/AACN Nurse Residency Program*. Retrieved from https://www.scha.org/files/jwillingham_vizient_nurse_residency.pdf

American Associaton of Colleges of Nursing. (2019). *Vizient/AACN Nurse Residency Program*. Retrieved from https://www.aacnnursing.org/Nurse-Residency-Program

Becher, J., & Visovsky, C. (2012). Horizontal violence in nursing. *Medsurg Nursing, 21*(4), 201–232. PMID:22966523

Center for Disease Control and Prevention. (2017). *Suicide risks and protective factors*. Retrieved from https://www.cdc.gov/violenceprevention/suicide/riskprotectivefactors.html

Chen, C., Lin, C., Wang, S., & Hou, T. (2009). A study of job stress, stress coping strategies, and job satisfaction for nurses working in middle-level operating rooms. *The Journal of Nursing Research, 17*(3), 199–210. doi:10.1097/JNR.0b013e3181b2557b PMID:19738448

Corbin, J., & Strauss, A. (2015). *Basics of qualitative research: Techniques and procedures for developing grounded theory* (4th ed.). Thousand Oaks, CA: Sage Publishing.

Cortina, L. M., Magley, V. J., Williams, J. H., & Laghout, R. D. (2001). Incivility in the workplace: Incidence and impact. *Journal of Occupational Health Psychology, 6*(1), 64–80. doi:10.1037/1076-8998.6.1.64 PMID:11199258

Davidson, J., Mendis, J., Stuck, A. R., DeMichele, G., & Zisook, S. (2018). Nurse suicide: Breaking the silence. In *National Academy of Medicine Perspectives*. Discussion Paper, National Academy of Medicine. Retrieved from https://nam.edu/nurse-suicide-breaking-the-silence

Federal Communications Commission. (2017). *Dial 211 for essential community services*. Retrieved from https://www.fcc.gov/consumers/guides/dial-211-essential-community-services

Institute of Medicine. (2003). *Keeping patients safe: Transforming the work environment for nurses*. Washington, DC: The National Academies Press.

Kang, J., Jeong, Y. J., & Kong, K. R. (2018). Threats to identity: A grounded theory approach on Student nurses' experience of incivility during clinical placement. *Journal of Korean Academy of Nursing*, *48*(1), 85–95. doi:10.4040/jkan.2018.48.1.85 PMID:29535287

Kanter, R. (1977). *Men and Women of the Corporation*. New York, NY: Basic Books.

Laschinger, H. K. S., Finegan, J. M., Shamian, J., & Wilk, P. (2001). Impact of structural and psychological empowerment on job strain in nursing work settings: Expanding Kanter's model. *The Journal of Nursing Administration*, *31*(5), 260–272. doi:10.1097/00005110-200105000-00006 PMID:11388162

McIntosh, W. L., Spies, E., Stone, D. M., Lokey, C. N., Trudeau, A. T., & Bartholow, B. (2016). Suicide Rates by Occupational Group — 17 States, 2012. *Centers for Disease Control and Prevention: Morbidity & Mortality Weekly Report*, *65*, 641–645. doi:10.15585/mmwr.mm6525a1 PMID:27359167

Moola, S., Ehlers, V. J., & Hattingh, S. P. (2008). Critical care nurses' perceptions of Stress and stress related situations in the workplace. *Curationis*, *31*(2), 74–83. doi:10.4102/curationis.v31i2.989 PMID:19006961

National Suicide Prevention Lifeline. (2018). *Talk to someone now*. Retrieved from https://suicidepreventionlifeline.org/

Oyeleye, O., Hanson, P., O'Connor, N., & Dunn, D. (2013). Relationship or workplace Incivility, stress, and burnout on nurses' turnover intentions and psychological Empowerment. *The Journal of Nursing Administration*, *43*(10), 536–542. doi:10.1097/NNA.0b013e3182a3e8c9 PMID:24061587

Quality and Safety Education for Nurses. (2019). *QSEN Competencies*. Retrieved from http://qsen.org/competencies/pre-licensure-ksas/

Reinhardt, T., Chavez, E., Jackson, M., & Mathews, W. C. (2005). Survey of physician well- being and health behaviors at an academic medical center. *Medical Education Online*, *10*(1), 4373. doi:10.3402/meo.v10i.4373 PMID:28253145

The American Nurse. (2016). *ANA calls for a culture of safety in all health care settings.* Retrieved from http://www.theamericannurse.org/index.php/2016/07/1Nurses2/ana-calls-for-a-culture-of-safety-in-all-health-care-settings

The Joint Commission. (2016). *Quick Safety 24: Bullying has no place in health care.* Retrieved from https://www.jointcommission.org/issues/article.aspx?Article=rFhOFvmOhideyaeaXWHwdF7iIsdGPTcEobEhA7d2RU=

Williams, S., & Cooper, C. L. (1998). Measuring occupational stress: Development of the pressure management indicator. *Journal of Occupational Health Psychology, 3*(4), 306–321. doi:10.1037/1076-8998.3.4.306 PMID:9805279

Windsor-Shellard, B. (2017). *Suicide by Occupation, England: 2011-2015.* Retrieved from https://www.ons.gov.uk/peoplepopulationandcommunity/birthsdeathsandmarriages/deaths/articles/suicidebyoccupation/england2011to2015#statistical-measures-of-suicide-by-occupation

Workplace Bullying Institute. (2014). *2014 WBI U.S. Workplace Bullying Survey February 2014.* Retrieved from http://www.workplacebullying.org/wbiresearch/wbi-2014-us-survey/

World Health Organization. (2018). *Mental health: Suicide data.* Retrieved from http://www.who.int/mental_health/prevention/suicide/suicideprevent/en/

Wu, S., Zhu, W., Wang, Z., & Lan, Y. (2007). Relationship between burnout and occupational stress among nurses in China. *Journal of Advanced Nursing, 59*(3), 233–239. doi:10.1111/j.1365-2648.2007.04301.x PMID:17590211

APPENDIX 1

Figure 2. Woman Untitled 2

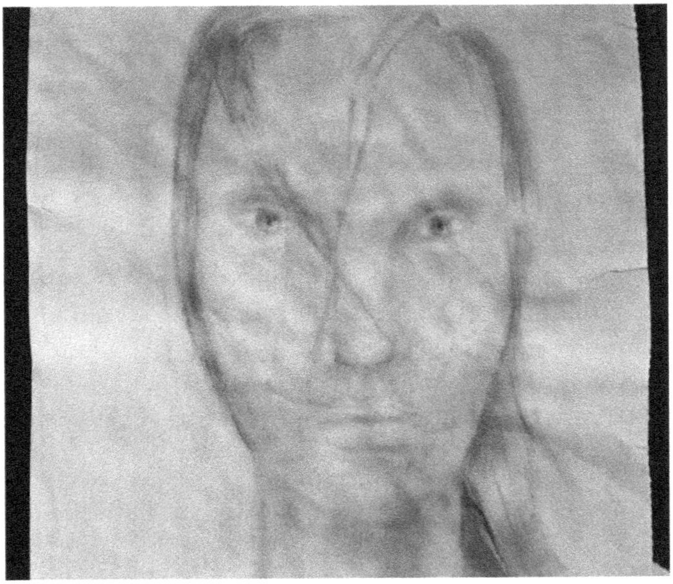

APPENDIX 2

Exploration Activities

Directions: The purpose of the *Exploration Activities* are to encourage reflection on the issue of uncivil conduct in nursing by recording one's feelings about the act of incivility. Please answer the questions or statements independently or within a group for discussion.

In your opinion, should health care facilities be more in-tuned to the problem of incivility within the profession of nursing?

____

Have you experienced job-related stress because of your interactions with an uncivil co-worker?

Are you currently experiencing job-related burnout?

Do you plan to leave a job that you have enjoyed in the past, because of your experience with incivility?

Do you feel that your decision to resign from a job that you enjoy because of a bully, is the wise choice to make at this time? If yes, why?

If you are currently being bullied in the workplace, have you disclosed to anyone what is happening to you and how it makes you feel?

Do you lose sleep at night replaying thoughts in your head regarding demeaning or stressful interactions you have had with someone that is intentionally bullying you at work?

Have you suffered headaches or stomach discomfort the moment you get to work in anticipation of a stressful day working with a co-worker that is unnecessarily rude or negative toward you?

Do you replay conversations of the uncivil behaviors of the person(s) whom is bullying you at work when you are driving home from work or when you are at home?

___

Have you spent valuable time with family and friends discussing the stress you are experiencing at work because of a bully?

___

Are you ready to disempower the negative effects that you have permitted the perpetrator(s) to have in your life?

___

___

Recognition that a bully exists solely because of their own insecurities, can lead to healing. Do you honestly feel that your bully is confident, or that their uncivil conduct is likely related to their own poor self-esteem and tendency to compare themselves to others?

___

___

___

___

___

Have you ever contemplated self-harm? If your answer is yes, it is important that you seek help. The decision to live is made when the realization that emotional pain and crises in life do not last forever. Dial 1-800-273-TALK, the National Suicide Prevention Lifeline for help.

___

___

Chapter 4
Suffering in Isolation

ABSTRACT

Unhealthy workplace environments have unfortunately been associated with the profession of nursing. Staffing shortages and long hours worked with high acuity patient caseloads can cause nursing professionals to feel overwhelmed, stressed, and anxious. Cultures of incivility can be accepted within some workplace environments as being normal. Nurse leaders that knowingly ignore patterns of disruptive behaviors by the nursing staff contribute to unit-based (and departmental) dysfunction. Perpetrators feel comfortable in continuing bullying behaviors because they have no fear of retribution. In these environments, nurse leaders themselves may engage in bullying and incivility behaviors. Chapter 4 provides nurses with instructions on how to report uncivil conduct that is not resolving and seek action against the perpetrator when mediation is not an option.

INTRODUCTION

Nurses experiencing bullying in the workplace can feel alone and isolated. It can be difficult for nurses to confide in their co-workers that they have been impacted by bullying by another nurse. Fear of being judged by others, may cause the affected nurse to not share their experience of being bullied. It is important for nurses affected by bullying to realize that they themselves are not weak and that incivility is not synonymous with a healthy workplace environment.

DOI: 10.4018/978-1-5225-7341-8.ch004

Shame can be a factor in the decision for nurses to maintain silence and isolate themselves when being bullied. Felblinger (2008) noted that some nurses tolerate uncivil conduct and do so without insight into their own pattern(s) of behavior. Perpetrators may utilize unacknowledged threats and attacks on their victim's self-esteem and self-worth in front of others as a means to promote shaming (Dzurec, Kennison, & Albataineh, 2014). The affected nurse, not responding to the perpetrator's attack, may inadvertently, give permission for the bullying to continue. Thus permitting incivility to remain in the workplace.

The toleration of unhealthy work environments has unfortunately been associated with the profession of nursing. Long hours and working short staffed while caring for patients with complex medical and surgical problems, can cause nurses to be frustrated and feel disempowered. Workplace violence can also affect nurses and other healthcare worker's safety, when co-workers, domestic partners, patients and patients' family members threaten physical harm to nurses working in health care environments (OSHA, 2016). Nurses must be provided education by their employers, on the dangers of not reporting incivility in the work environment, so that they are empowered to protect themselves and other nurses from harm.

Cultures of Incivility

Within workplaces with cultures of incivility, bullying is tolerated and viewed as the norm. Persons who report bullying in these workplaces are treated as if they are a part of the problem and not the solution. It is important that victims of bullying realize that bullying occurring over a period of time, for example, over a year, is not an issue of perception, but one of deliberate targeting of a person or persons with the intention of emotional or physical harm.

When victims of incivility are working within workplaces that tolerate cultures of incivility, it is important to understand that when incidences of bullying are reported, these incidences should be documented in writing. The latter establishes a distinct pattern of incivility. Any persons that observed the bullying should be included in investigations. Although difficult to recall the events of bullying, nurses that are victims can potentially create a dialogue within workplace cultures that have in the past, chosen to ignore issues of incivility.

Following the Chain of Command

When affected by workplace incivility, it is imperative that the chain of command be followed with notification of a direct supervisor first. Whenever possible, attempt to clarify or set boundaries with the perpetrator to maintain a professional relationship. If the perpetrator is not receptive to resolution of the problem, if in fact there is an identified issue, then the affected nurse should speak with a supervisor.

The purpose of the nurse meeting with a supervisor is to facilitate discussion regarding the uncivil behavior from the perpetrator, with the hope of mediation occurring in the presence of the supervisor, between the affected nurse and the perpetrator. The goal of this meeting is to see if resolution is possible with the mediation, and also to provide a different perspective on the nurse-to-nurse issues with uncivil conduct from a person that is familiar with both parties. If this does not occur, or if the supervisor is in alliance with the perpetrator(s), then the affected nurse should make an appointment to meet with a representative from Human Resources.

Human Resources

The Department of Human Resources (HR) is in charge of the hiring and training of personnel that are employed within an organization (HRRO, 2018). Administratively, HR serves as a resource for employees to maintain awareness of their employee rights, opportunities for changes and growth in career paths, benefits (i.e. insurance, tuition reimbursement, retirement, etc.) and expectations of work culture, dress code, and acceptable behavioral conduct within the workplace. HR also serves as a liaison between the employee and the employer.

For nurses meeting with HR to discuss an issue with incivility, an appointment to meet with a representative should occur only after the nurse or nurses has met with their supervisor. The initial meeting with HR is for gathering information and the nurse(s) requesting consultation on how to best resolve and or cope with the uncivil conduct. After the initial meeting, as long as the nurse feels that there is no potential for harm by the perpetrator, the nurse may decide to resolve the issue on their own applying the information provided by HR.

Nurses who do not find resolution with information and support provided by HR in dealing with nurse-to-nurse workplace incivility, may make a formal complaint with an HR representative, against the perpetrator. If the affected nurse makes the decision to make a formal complaint, anecdotal notes describing situations when the bullying occurred that includes: actual dates, times the events occurred, details of the event, and whom was involved or witnessed the event, should be shared. This information is necessary to substantiate the validity of the formal complaint.

Issues with Mediation

It is important that nurses affected by incivility realize that a formal mediation performed by an HR representative involves two parties signing a confidential agreement regarding the discussion of the problem at hand. In this case, both parties are acknowledging participation in the disagreement or dispute. The problem in using HR mediation agreements is that in bullying, one person or persons is being targeted and often targeted in a situation that was unprovoked by them. The perpetrator and the bullied victim in no way have the same experience. A concern with workplaces that encourage this practice, is that victims of bullying can be further victimized during the mediation process, as perpetrators attempt to assume the role of victim themselves to avoid potential disciplinary action.

Labor Unions

The purpose of a labor union is to represent employees in the improvement of work conditions, benefits, contractual violations or provisions, wage bargaining, disputes at the managerial level, and overall improvement of working conditions. Labor unions are not present in every health care facility. Nurses that work in facilities with unions and are paying membership fees, should meet with a union representative to develop an understanding of how their specific union has benefited employees currently and in the past. Also, inquire if they can assist with your specific problem with bullying. If not, then consider the necessity of further investigation occurring alternatively by hiring legal counsel with a specialization within employment law. If the organization has a Diversity Officer at that their facility, a request can be made to meet with the Diversity Officer to discuss workplace-related concerns. Diversity Officers uphold the United States Equal Opportunity Commission's (EEOC) employment practices and are knowledgeable about employee rights and organizational policies and regulations within the institutions in which they are employed (National Association of Diversity Officers in Higher Education, 2019).

Understanding the Equal Employment Opportunity Commission Prohibited Practices

The United States Equal Opportunity Commission prohibited employment practices include: discrimination against someone because of their genetic information, disability, age (40 or older), sex (i.e. pregnancy, gender identity, and sexual orientation), race, national origin, color, religion, and disability (EEOC, 2018). If a nurse believes that he or she fits these discriminatory categories with regard to the reason that uncivil conduct has been directed toward them, the nurse may consider contacting an attorney that specializes in employment law or discussing their concerns with their employer's Diversity Officer (if the role exists within the organization). Consultation with an employment law attorney (an attorney that consults on cases involving work-related legal disputes) can help nurses affected by incivility, to decipher whether discrimination may be involved and if the uncivil behaviors are in violation of the EEOC.

Figure 1. Reporting uncivil conduct

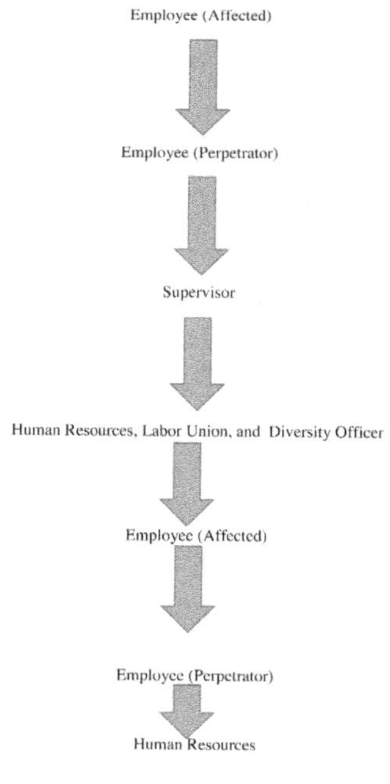

Reporting incivility in the workplace can be very anxiety provoking for nurses. While nurses are aware that they have been negatively impacted by bullying, there is a normal desire to not disrupt the work environment by casting blame on the perpetrator(s) of the act. Figure 1 can assist nurses in the reporting of uncivil conduct within the work environment.

Unresolved Uncivil Conduct

After the affected nurse has attempted to resolve the issue with the perpetrator without resolution, the nurse should notify their manager or supervisor. If there is no resolution found at this stage, then HR should be notified so that some form of mediation can occur to attempt to resolve the situation. If indicated, HR will further investigate the situation. If the bullying persists after the latter interventions, the affected nurse may consider consulting an employment law attorney. Figure 2 assists the nurse in dealing with unresolved uncivil conduct.

Case Study 7 is a hypothetical case study and all characters are fictional. In this case study, Benjamin and Hank are nurses that are peers with a history of attending nursing school together and working on the same clinical unit.

Figure 2. Unresolved uncivil conduct

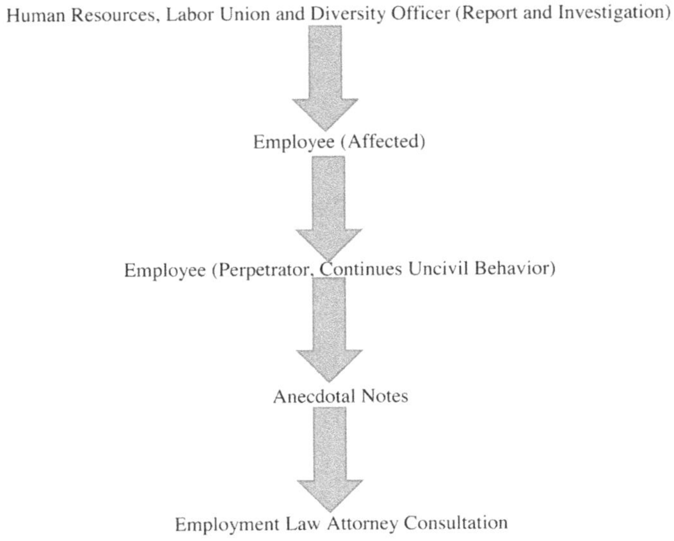

Case Study 7: Benjamin and Hank

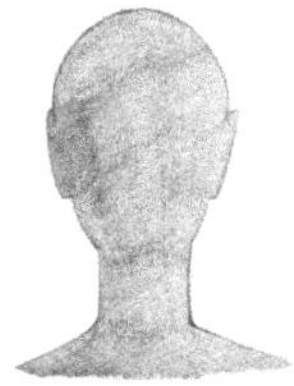

Benjamin and Hank have been friends since nursing school. The two co-workers are employed by the same hospital and work on the same clinical unit. Benjamin and Hank's collegiality and team collaboration with others on the unit, were notable strengths that the two co-workers consistently demonstrated among their peers, patients, and nurse manager.

Hank started dating one of the nurses on the unit. The nurse Hank dated was a devout Rastafarian who wore dreadlocks in her hair. Hank, within seven months of dating this nurse, began to dread his medium length hair.

Hank later converted to Rastafarianism. His time with Benjamin was limited, as he frequently would go to the hospital chapel to pray alone on his breaks. Benjamin approached Hank one day when they were both leaving work and walking to the parking garage. He asked Hank why he had converted to the Rastafarian faith. Benjamin confided that he missed their friendship. Hank abruptly ended the conversation and proceeded to walk to his car.

The nurse manager, four days after Benjamin's conversation with Hank asked to speak privately with Benjamin. Hank had made a complaint against Benjamin to the Human Resource Department. The complaint alleged that Benjamin had discriminated against his co-worker based on his religious beliefs.

Is Benjamin the Victim Here?

Benjamin did not demonstrate discriminatory behaviors toward Hank based on his religion. He appropriately approached his co-worker as they departed the clinical unit and entered the parking garage. Benjamin inquired as to why Hank had converted to Rastafarianism, but did not criticize nor harass him because of his religious belief. Hence, Benjamin was wrongfully accused.

Be Aware of What You Are Communicating

Nurses must be aware of their verbal and nonverbal communication in the workplace. In absence of malice, Benjamin inquired about his co-worker's decision to convert. When his co-worker chose to end the conversation, no further attempts were made by Benjamin reengage the conversation. This does not constitute incivility.

Not All Disagreements Are Incivility

Workplaces are professional environments. Failure to treat others respectfully in the workplace, could potentially lead to negative sanctions. When experiencing issues with communication with a colleague, seek resolution via a neutral party mediating or preferably, attempt to calmly address the person yourself. Unresolved conflicts will eventually manifest themselves behaviorally, because no resolution has occurred. The strain in Hank and Benjamin's relationship likely was a result of Hank's conversion, and could be resolved with mediation at the nurse manager level only if affecting their work relationship. Given that a formal complaint was made by Hank to Human Resources, it is necessary for Benjamin to meet with a Human Resources representative and address the complaint. The HR representative will then investigate the complaint and provide remediation.

Diversity and Inclusion

Healthy workplaces are those that foster respect for diversity and inclusion. These workplaces offer trainings that educate employees about working peaceably with co-workers of different racial and ethnic backgrounds, genders, cultures, political, and religious beliefs. Miller and Katz (2010) define inclusion as, "a sense of belonging: feeling respected, valued, and seen for who we are as individuals; and a level of supportive energy and commitment from leaders, colleagues, and others so that we- collectively and individually- can do our best work" (p. 437). When people collectively learn to view others in absence of presumption(s) and prejudices, relationships have the opportunity to develop and flourish.

There will be situations in the workplace whereby education of employees and employers about differences can resolve ineffective communication patterns that do not constitute incivility, nor bullying. Creating workplace cultures that foster comfort in communicating about diversity, such as race and cultural differences, can reinforce the value of healthy workplaces. Also, educating nursing staff on the value of conflict management, by intruding techniques that can be used to reframe conflict as being a positive way to resolve differences, can be beneficial for employees in learning to deescalate situations (Choudhary, 2018). Additionally, by placing priority on healthy work environments and adopting a zero tolerance (ANA, 2015) for uncivil conduct, organizations can decrease bullying and incivility. Organizations adopting formal codes of conduct that do not permit incivility or bullying in the workplace (Schmidt, MacWilliams, & Neal-Boylan, 2017) can reinforce compliance with zero tolerance of bullying and incivility, by requiring all employees to sign compliance documents.

Appendix 1 contains exploration activities that address discrimination within the workplace. Ineffective communication is examined as a way in which misinterpretation can mask that which is not uncivil behavior in the workplace. Bullying and incivility being involved in exclusionary behaviors is explored.

REFERENCES

American Nurses Association. (2015). Zero tolerance. *The American Nurse*, *47*(5), 1–11. PMID:26563037

Choudhary, L. (2018). Educational strategies for conflict management. *Nursing*, *48*(12), 14–15. doi:10.1097/01.NURSE.0000547734.74555.3c PMID:30461703

Dzurec, L. C., Kennison, M., & Albataineh, R. (2014). Unacknowledged threats proferred "in a Manner of speaking": Recognizing workplace bullying as shaming. *Journal of Nursing Scholarship*, *46*(4), 281–291. doi:10.1111/jnu.12080 PMID:24754642

Felblinger, D. M. (2008). Incivility and bullying in the workplace and nurses' shame responses. *Journal of Obstetric, Gynecologic, and Neonatal Nursing*, *37*(2), 234–242. doi:10.1111/j.1552-6909.2008.00227.x PMID:18336449

Human Resources Research Organization. (2018). *Who we are*. Retrieved from https://www.humrro.org/corpsite/landing-page/what-we-do

Miller, F. A., & Katz, J. H. (2010). Inclusion: The HOW for organizational breakthrough. In *Practicing organization development: A guide for leading change* (3rd ed.; pp. 436–445). San Francisco, CA: Pfeiffer Publishing.

National Association of Diversity Officers in Higher Education. (2019). *Standards of Professional Practice for Chief Diversity Officers.* Retrieved from https://www.nadohe.org/standards-of-professional-practice-for-chief-diversity-officers

Rainford, W.C., Wood, S., McMullen, P.C., Philipsen, N.D. (n.d.). The disruptive force of lateral violence in the health care setting. *Journal of Nursing Practice, 11*(2), 157–164.

Schmidt, B. J., MacWilliams, B. R., & Neal-Boylan, L. (2017). Becoming inclusive: A Code of conduct for inclusion and diversity. *Journal of Professional Nursing*, *33*(2), 102–107. doi:10.1016/j.profnurs.2016.08.014 PMID:28363383

United States Department of Labor Occupational Safety and Health Administration. (2016). *Association position statement on incivility, bullying, and workplace violence. Federal Register, 81*(235), 88147-88167. Retrieved from https://www.osha.gov/sites/default/files/laws-regs/federalregister/2016-12-07.pdf

United States Equal Employment Opportunity Commission. (2018). *Prohibited Employment Policies/Practices.* Retrieved from https://www.eeoc.gov//laws/practices/

APPENDIX 1

Exploration Activities

Directions: The purpose of the *Exploration Activities* are to encourage reflection on the issue of uncivil conduct in nursing by recording one's feelings about the act of incivility.

Were you familiar with the EEOC prohibited practices in the workplace prior to reading this chapter?

____

____

____

____

____

____

Have you ever been discriminated against within the workplace?

____

____

____

____

____

Have you ever observed a colleague being discriminated against in the workplace?

____

____

____

____

____

____

____

How do you think it feels to be discriminated against?

____
____
____
____
____
____

Do you believe Benjamin was intentionally discriminating against Hank's Rastafarian religion?

____
____
____
____
____
____

Can you identify comments made by Benjamin about his co-worker Hank that could have been interpreted as being discriminatory?

____
____
____
____
____
____

How could this alleged act of discrimination by Benjamin toward Hank have been avoided?

____
____
____
____
____
____

Did Benjamin engage in workplace incivility?

Chapter 5
Beyond the Pain

ABSTRACT

Healthy workplaces promote inclusionary behaviors. When nurses experience exclusionary behaviors such as bullying and incivility, there may also be hidden issues with acceptance of diversity in the workplace environment. Educating nursing staff on the importance of variations in age, culture, gender, sex, race, ethnicity, and religion in the workplace can help facilitate communication among staff. For example, organizations can use educational forums to discuss how different cultures vary in the addressing of conflict within the workplace; some cultures may prefer to reach consensus rather than be confrontational. Chapter 5 discusses strategies that nurses and organizations can implement, such as Team Strategies and Tools to Enhance Performance and Patient Safety (TeamSTEPPS). TeamSTEPPS is a curriculum that can be used to improve teamwork skills, communication, and build team collaboration.

INTRODUCTION

The profession of nursing in itself can be challenging. Nurses provide care to people in different settings (i.e. home care, clinics, inpatient units, etc.) and stabilize patients with complex disease processes, while collaborating within a team of other health care professionals (Chen, Lin, Wang, & Hou, 2009). Nurses work within rapid-paced health care environments that can be stressful. Therefore, having to cope with the additional stress of incivility from a co-worker, can be overwhelming.

DOI: 10.4018/978-1-5225-7341-8.ch005

Recognizing the Effects of Incivility

It is important for nurses to be aware of the signs and symptoms of uncivil behaviors within the workplace, so that they can be readily addressed. Repeated exposure, for example, to condescending language, criticism, and superficial listening, can cause the nurse to feel disempowered and disconnected. The latter impacting job satisfaction and productivity. The pain of working in an environment that does not value your contributions or you as a person, can lead to mental and physical illness.

Social bullying is defined as an experiential and behavioral phenomenon. Nurses affected by social bullying experience intimidation, persistent criticism, insults, abuses of power used against them, and malicious behavior. Wieland and Beitz (2015) conducted a qualitative phenomenological study on nurses' resilience to social bullying occurring within academia. Seventeen nursing faculty that were self-identified as having experienced bullying in the workplace, were audiotaped as they shared their stories. There were three distinct chronologic periods that led to a theme in the interviews. These three chronologic periods were identified as being *during bullying, decisional phase, and after bullying* (Wieland & Beitz, 2015).

The 17 nursing faculty that participated in the Wieland and Beitz study recalled enduring cultures whereby bullying was accepted, as were cyberbullying, and power and control issues. The uncivil behavior was often perpetrated by senior faculty and administrators. The affected nursing faculty found that once they began to recognize patterns of bullying and no longer rationalized that the bullying was normal to the field of academia, that they became resilient. With this insight came the ability of each faculty participant, to better understand how their work environments functioned, and how to manage their own personal responses to the bullying experience.

According to Wieland and Beitz (2015), in discussing the commonalities of the 17 resilient faculty that experienced workplace bullying, "In becoming aware of bullying and sharing this awareness with colleagues, participants began to set personal boundaries to avoid abuse. They also observed colleagues' strategies and learned them. Participants reported using physical and mental strategies, talking with colleagues, and faculty and student teaching evaluations to buttress self-worth" (p. 291). Self-conscious decisions to no longer tolerate the mental abuse of the perpetrators, caused these faculty to successfully remain in their positions and flourish. Limitations of this study were that there were no minority faculty interviewed. Participants were 95% female and 85% white. Therefore bullying within the context of discrimination could not be evaluated.

Diversity and Positive Work Environments

Schmidt, MacWilliams, and Neal-Boylan (2017) noted that exclusionary behaviors in the profession of nursing are an increasing concern. Nurses that experience bullying, workplace violence, and incivility are likely according to Schmidt, MacWilliam, and Neal-Boylan, experiencing exclusionary behaviors. Inclusivity embraces differences and are conducive to workplace environments that have a zero tolerance for nurse-to-nurse incivility and bullying.

Organizations that seek to educate nurses on the importance of diversity in the workplace such as with religion, race, culture, ethnicity, gender, and age, facilitate communication on differences. In the facilitating of conversations about diversity, organizations promote inclusion via the valuing of differences. For example, health care organizations can implement educational forums on topics such as nurses of different ages and generations engaging in conversations about different approaches to patient care and perceived work ethics. Hence, the opportunity to foster healthier work environments.

Building Healthy Healthcare Teams

Team Strategies and Tools to Enhance Performance and Patient Safety (TeamSTEPPS) is a curriculum that health care organizations can implement to improve teamwork skills and communication. The curriculum is evidenced-based and uses case studies (in varied health care settings, i.e. outpatient clinics, long-term care) and current health care research findings to help health care professionals respectfully interact and maintain workplace environments conducive to patients receiving safe quality health care (Agency for Healthcare Research and Quality, 2019). Outcome driven, the TeamSTEPPS training provides nurses and other healthcare professionals with knowledge about how behavior can affect co-workers and patients.

TeamSTEPPS strategies can be incorporated into simulations in health care environments and in academia, to train nurses and prelicensure student nurses on the importance of team collaboration. The TeamSTEPPS curriculum includes PowerPoints (TeamSTEPPS, 2019) with learning objectives, scenarios and instructional tools in developing a simulation. Levels of simulation analysis can be constructed to address the learning needs of different healthcare professionals (i.e. nurses, physicians, physician assistants, advanced practice registered nurses, or respiratory therapist) and the actual clinical setting (i.e. a medical unit, neonatal intensive care unit, or operating room).

Seeking Counseling or Therapy

In deciding to see a counselor or therapist, the nurse should be aware that a counselor tends to be someone that is certified or licensed to provide support or guidance to persons experiencing problems (i.e. substance abuse counselor, recovery programs) and may have a bachelor's or associate degree. Whereas, a therapist is more likely to have a master's or doctorate degree and be skilled in providing individual, family, or couple's therapy. Nurses deciding to seek the help of a counselor or therapist, may want to start with a visit to their primary care provider or their employee assistance program for consultation.

The experience of bullying can be psychologically damaging. Nurses affected by bullying have been exposed to persistent negative words said about them and negative acts perpetrated against them, that were unprovoked. Nurses may ask themselves why they were targeted, and what about their personality drove a person or persons to target them. The realization that a bully or bullies target others because of their own insecurities, must be made by the affected nurse. Nurses can benefit from seeking the assistance of a counselor or therapist to understand their bullying experience and to be empowered to change the situation by protecting themselves and others.

A counselor or therapist can provide an objective view of the nurse's circumstance and how the bully has established a predictable pattern of attack. Bullies will typically, strategize their psychological (or physical) attacks based upon the affected nurse's response to their acts of uncivil behavior. When the affected nurse, with the assistance of the counselor or therapist, can recognize when the perpetrator is more likely to demonstrate uncivil behavior, the affected nurse can counter the attack by directly addressing the bully and the negative responses, or simply ignoring the comments and the bully themselves. Hence, disempowering the bully (or bullies).

Nurses can also use therapy or counseling to explore their own sense of self-worth and value within their work environment and personal lives. With a counselor or therapist, nurses can also address histories of abuse and neglect that may contribute to their tolerance of incivility. The goal of therapy and counseling is to strengthen the nurse and return wholeness and resiliency during and after bullying has occurred.

Treating Medical Problems

Nurses that experience physical problems associated with being bullied such as gastrointestinal problems and headaches, should see a healthcare provider to rule-out stress-related illness versus the presence of an actual disease process(es). It is important that nurses share with their healthcare provider, their situation of being bullied and how they are coping or not coping. Healthcare providers can help persons being bullied by referring them to a counselor or therapist and focusing their own assessments on the maintenance of the health of the affected person. For example, a physiological response to bullying could be an elevation in pulse and blood pressure related to stress and anxiety. A healthcare provider can help the nurse monitor these objective findings and suggest ways of reducing stress such as exercise and eating healthy while the problem of bullying is being addressed in therapy or counseling sessions.

Decision to Stay or Leave the Job

The decision to leave a job must be made by the nurse when there is no support in the workplace for resolution of the bullying problem, the nurse feels unsafe or physically threatened, or when the health of the nurse is becoming compromised. If the nurse feels that he or she is committed to and enjoys the job, then the interventions of healthcare, therapy and counseling, and working within the institution to write a formal complaint against the perpetrator, must be implemented as soon as possible.

Nurses must remember, that they do not have to tolerate uncivil behavior. Incivility is unprofessional conduct that negatively impacts the nurse and the patients the nurse provides care to. If the nurse is in academia, their ability to teach and conduct research necessary to attain tenure, is impaired. Nurses must make the decision to disempower workplace bullies and expose their uncivil behaviors. In doing so, in clinical settings, patients are potentially unharmed and in academia, future nurses are mentored to learn to respect one another.

Work-Life Balance

Raja, Javed, and Abbas (2017) examined how workplace bullying can manifest in work-family conflict when correlated with job burnout. Raja et al., studied 151 full-time employees applying 3-wave time lagged field data.

Workplace bullying was measured using the Negative Acts Questionnaire (NAQ; Einarsen & Raknes, 1997), an 8-item (1, never to 5, daily) addressing exposure to different situations of victimization and bullying. A 5-item scale (1, strongly disagree to 5, strongly agree) was used to measure Work-Family Conflict (WFC; Netemeyer, Boles, & McMurrian, 1996). An example of a question item would be, "*the demands of my work interfered with my home and family life.*" Lastly, Job Burnout (JB; Demerouti & Nachreiner, 1998) was measured using an 8-item scale. States of physical exhaustion, feeling overtaxed from work, and the necessity for rest, were examined. An example of an item statement would be "*after my work, I regularly feel worn out and weary.*"

The results of the Raja et al. (2017) study were that there was a relationship between workplace bullying and work-family conflict. These findings suggested that workers whom experience bullying are more likely to have an imbalance in their personal lives and experience burnout. In order for workers to protect themselves from burnout that impacts their life at home, the workplace bullying must end.

Huntington, et al. (2011) conducted a qualitative study with 7,604 nurses from the United Kingdom, Australia, and New Zealand examining the health of nurses, workforce characteristics, and work-life balance. Of the 7,604 nurses participating in the study, 1,909 submitted 162 qualitative comments that were analyzed and arranged into four themes. These themes include: *organizational (non) care* raising the seemingly lack of support from management; *embodied care* which discussed the impact on nurses' emotional and physical health; *(un)collegial self-care,* the origin of professional and bullying relationships; and *quality/quantity care* addressing nurses' ability to provide quality care with increased pressures of work.

Nurses participating within the Huntington et al. (2011) study identified issues such as job-related stress, work-place injuries, working with nurses not well-qualified nor stable in performing the job, and bullying, affecting the health of nurses. Results indicated that while the latter issues are not new to the nursing profession, there remains a gap in nursing between theory and practice. When nurses experience work-life imbalance, retention of nurses within the workplace can be difficult (Huntington et al., 2011; Raja et al., 2017).

Case Study 8 is a hypothetical case study and all characters are fictional. In this case study, Ellen, a nurse educator, experiences bullying and incivility within the academic setting.

Case Study 8: Ellen

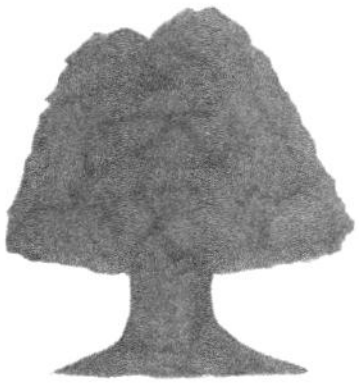

Ellen Peterson has been a nurse educator at a four-year private university for five years. Ellen's work with the nursing students has been exemplary. Her changes to the curriculum had improved students' performance on key components of the National Council Licensure Exam (NCLEX-RN) for registered nurses and her classroom evaluations from students were reflective of students' continuous growth in their studies. Nursing students who took her classes reported being academically challenged, having an increase in clinical and critical thinking, and an ability to apply theory to the bedside care of medically and surgically complex patients.

Ellen recently co-authored two nursing textbooks and published three articles. However, as she readily approached tenure, she questioned her desire to continue to teach within a nursing program. It seemed no matter how hard she worked, fault was always found in her efforts. Ellen was ridiculed in department meetings and almost daily, bullied by her peers.

The taunting in meetings was normalized by the other faculty as a means to be initiated into the department. However, it seemed for a select few faculty that had been at the school for over seven years, the taunting had never ended. Ellen believed, like her colleagues, she too could withstand the name calling and the demeaning comments that challenged her intellect, but it proved too much over time. One day, as Ellen was walking toward her office, she collapsed in the hallway.

Ellen was rushed to the hospital by ambulance where she was diagnosed with a myocardial infarction (heart attack). The diagnosis was shocking to Ellen, she had no risk factors. Her cholesterol levels were normal, she exercised five times a week, and did not have high blood pressure, diabetes or any underlying cardiac issues. Ellen was happily married to a supportive spouse for 30 years and had two grown daughters. The only identifiable stress in Ellen's life was her job as a nurse educator.

Ellen Goes to Therapy

Four weeks after her heart attack, Ellen began seeing a therapist. She was very tearful and worried that she may not be able to work as a nurse again. She shared with the therapist, "From the time I was nine years old, I always wanted to be a nurse. What if I cannot return to work?" The therapist assured Ellen that it was likely that she could return to being a nurse, but would require support to do so.

During sessions with the therapist, Ellen shared stories of patients she had cared for, the progression of her career and why she had decided to become a nurse educator. Ellen was passionate about her nursing career and saw it as a vocation, not just a job. She seemed dumbfounded that her colleagues would intentionally treat her disrespectfully when she was working collaboratively with them with the mutual goal of helping nursing students excel.

Something to Consider

The therapist asked Ellen to begin to journal to reveal unconscious and conscious thoughts she may have never processed while being bullied. Ellen began to write daily in her journal. Ellen seldom expressed feeling of anger and frustration in her journal writings. The therapist was concerned and asked Ellen did she harbor any negative feelings toward her bullies. Ellen shared that she had difficulty becoming outwardly angry.

The therapist asked Ellen, "What if a nurse was telling a patient with diabetes during a family meeting that they "just didn't measure up when it came to managing their diabetes." However, the patient's blood glucose levels ranged between 99 mg/dL to 101mg/dL daily, the patient exercised 5 days a week and closely monitored their carbohydrate intake? The therapist then inquired, "Ellen, what would be your response to this nurse?" Ellen instantly began to advocate on behalf of the patient and how she would reassure the patient that they were managing their diabetes very well. "That nurse, said Ellen, is totally wrong. Clinically and logically what the nurse said, makes no sense."

This was Ellen's aha moment. She stared at the therapist quietly and nodded her head. "What my co-workers have done to me makes no sense. I have been doing the right thing. I arrive at work and do my job well. I engage my students in the learning process and I thoroughly research current clinical practice guidelines. I am published in textbooks and journals and speak nationally. I am always professional and respectful to my colleagues and the student nurses."

Ellen then shared, "I was bullied for no good reason! I am the one who is sick now!" Tearful, she sat quietly for 10 minutes. Ellen then left the office informing the therapist that she would call to make a follow up appointment.

Two weeks past and the therapist attempted five times to call Ellen by phone. Ellen did not respond until three weeks later. Ellen explained that in the last session she felt "too vulnerable and emotionally exposed." Ellen spoke on the phone for about 15 minutes with the therapist about how she felt and planned the next steps for the continuation of her therapy.

The therapist and Ellen resumed sessions and met every-other-week. During their sessions, Ellen shared a written plan that she had worked on at home on her own. The plan listed the positives and negatives of remaining within her current faculty position. For Ellen, the list contained the answer specific to her needs and no one else's. Ellen decided to resign from her faculty position.

The Transition

Ellen continued therapy after submitting her resignation and beginning her search for new employment. She returned to clinical nursing as an associate director of nursing at a rehabilitation hospital. She was so excited when she received the job offer. Ellen has learned to enjoy life and not allow others to dictate her happiness within the workplace. She has also become an advocate for nurses in addressing workplace violence and incivility through writing articles, presenting on the topic nationally, and teaching newly hired nurses at the healthcare facility at which she is employed, the danger of nurse-to-nurse bullying.

Beginning Again

Ellen learned that it is never too late to begin again, especially when one's health has been compromised. Because incivility can effect nurses' mental and physical health, it is imperative that the bullying be addressed early to avoid the potential negative consequences of poor health outcomes. Nurses must give themselves permission to say *no more* to bullying in the workplace and to seek assistance in ending workplace incivility.

Case Study 9 is a hypothetical case study and all characters are fictional. In this case study, John, a critical care nurse, decides to become a nurse manager and experiences bullying and incivility within the clinical setting.

Case Study 9: John

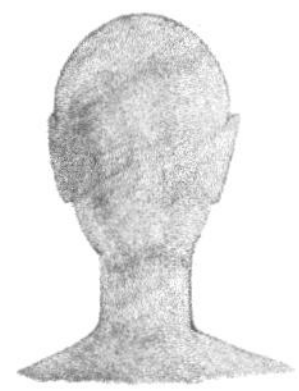

John is a single father of two children, a son and a daughter. His wife died 6 years ago of a brain aneurysm. Since his wife's death, John has managed his career as a critical care nurse and a full-time father well. John's teenage son and daughter frequently share with others that their dad is their best friend and always calm in a crisis and supportive.

With his children getting older and his son, the oldest child, going to college next year, John decided to apply for a managerial position in a newly opened critical care unit at his job. The extra money that came with the managerial position, could help with paying for college tuition. John interviewed and was offered the position of nurse manager.

The hours spent at work were long, as John began to acclimate himself to his new job. John was assigned a mentor to help him with transitioning from the staff nurse role, to nursing management. His mentor was a nurse manager who also worked in the same healthcare system, but on a different campus.

John's mentor, Bridget, was a great support to him. She like John, had worked several years in critical care before becoming a nurse manager. As a mentor, Bridget was always readily available to help John with dealing with the development of a unit budget plan to present to administration, displaying data related to initiatives such as the reduction of central line-associated bloodstream infections (CLABSI), and using the electronic scheduling system to schedule all unit staff. In their healthcare system, their units were the top performing critical care units with high patient satisfaction survey results and health outcomes data for patients that were reflective of a reduction in patient length of stays.

Something Changed

One year had quickly passed and John was very comfortable performing his job as a nurse manager. He began to gradually reduce his long work hours to spend more time with his children and spent less time with his mentor Bridget. Bridget would come by his office for unplanned visits.

One evening, when John was working late in his office planning the schedule for summer vacation coverage for the unit, Bridget visited. The visit was unplanned and John was very busy and trying to finish his work so that he could attend a sporting event at his daughter's school. John explained why he was in a rush to leave work to Bridget, but Bridget shared that she needed to talk about a problem on her unit. John was thankful to Bridget for all that she had done to help him with orienting to his new role, so he stayed and listened.

Three hours later, John arrived home late and his daughter was in tears about his having missed her school event. She had been transported home by her older brother. John felt guilty and overwhelmed. Over the course of two months, Bridget repeated this pattern of delaying John at work at least three times. By the fourth time, John was abrupt and informed Bridget that he had to prioritize the needs of his children over work. Bridget reluctantly agreed. It was after this encounter that John began to see a change in their relationship.

Rejection Not Taken Well

Bridget was very upset. She felt that John had taken advantage of her, and the knowledge she shared as his mentor. She could not believe this had happened again with a male colleague. She mentored them, provided support and once they learned the job, her services were not needed. She was dismissed. Bridget promised herself that she would make certain this never happened again.

Bridget went to speak with the director of her service line. She informed the director that John was verbally abusive to her. Bridget shared that she feared for her safety given his inappropriate and disruptive behavior in the workplace. The director responded swiftly, informing Human Resources (HR) and John's service line director on his campus. Within 24-hours, John was asked to report to the HR Department where he met with his service line director and a representative from HR.

John was dumbfounded when asked to come to HR. His first response was to inquire if there was an issue with one of his nursing staff. When his service line director and the HR representative explained the reason he was asked to meet with them, John was shocked. He denied having done anything to harm Bridget. He explained that the long hours of work at his new job, had impacted the time he spent with his children. Bridget's unplanned visits to his office impeded him from getting home to his family.

The Investigation

The service line director and HR representative informed John that an investigation would occur and that this may involve interviewing staff and other witnesses. John readily agreed. He knew that he was innocent. The investigation went on for four weeks, as Bridget continued to complain that John called her at work. No evidence was found. The initial investigation focused on verbal harassment and was dismissed.

Six months later, one of the nurses on John's unit shared with HR that John had poor social skills and was abrupt in his communications with her. This nurse had documented days and times of inappropriate interactions with John. The documented incidences centered on John asking her to work extra shifts to cover the unit staffing needs. John was again summoned to HR to meet with his service line director and an HR representative. He was frustrated and felt betrayed. When asked why he thought he was asked to come to HR John, stated, "More lies, and I did nothing."

John was informed during the meeting in HR that he would have to take one week of paid leave given that this was the second complaint of his being verbally inappropriate. John agreed and after having a meeting with staff, took a week off. While at home, HR called John and asked him not to return to work for an additional week and that he would not be paid.

A Disturbance in Work-Life Balance

While at home, John could not sleep and his appetite was poor. Arguments with his teenage son and daughter were almost daily. John was frightened that he would lose his job. He could not believe that the lies of two co-workers could be supported in absence of solid evidence. John, after discussing his concerns with his church pastor, decided to seek the advice of an employment law attorney.

The employment law attorney informed John that he was likely being bullied at work. The attorney informed John that he did not believe that the complaints by the two employees would lead to John's termination. He recommended that John await the completion of the HR investigation. John took the attorney's advice.

John returned to work, however the complaints continued from both his former mentor Bridget and the staff nurse on his unit. John, tired of the unsubstantiated complaints, decided to resign. One evening, as John was packing the contents within his office, a nurse assistant requested to speak with him. The nurse assistant shared that she had overheard a staff nurse talking on the phone about "Screwing you over." The nurse assistant said to John, "I think you are being set up about something. I am not sure what, but you may want to investigate this."

Deception Can Happen in Health Care

John called the attorney he met with and discussed what the nurse assistant had reported to him. The attorney, in collaboration with John, secured the services of a private investigator. However, the day before the private investigator was to observe the staff nurse, one of the registered nurses on John's unit contacted HR and informed them that Bridget and the staff nurse were conspiring against John to get him fired. The basis of their plan was Bridget having felt rejected by John.

The service line director and HR representative met with John and he was provided his lost income and an apology regarding the bullying he experienced in the workplace. The staff nurse and Bridget received disciplinary action and both employees ultimately resigned. John was emotionally traumatized by what had occurred and its impact on his home life. John and his children, decided to attend family therapy to mend their strained relationships.

The Many Forms of Bullying

John's bullies used falsehoods and misrepresentation of facts to attempt to undermine him. As a male, he was vulnerable for potentially being labelled as aggressive in his interactions with his female colleagues. It is important that males are well aware of the presence of bullying in the workplace and how there can potentially be a fine line between bullying and harassment.

If accused of inappropriate communication by co-workers, victims should begin to record daily, anecdotal notes and avoid meeting people alone in the workplace. Immediately communicate your suspicions to your supervisor so it is documented. It may help to share your suspicions with a trusted co-worker, so that you are not alone in what you are experiencing. Notify HR and an immediate supervisor of the bullying.

Examining John's Story

John was not in any way at fault for how Bridget handled her perceived feelings of rejection. Her feelings were long-standing and likely a reaction to issues that occurred in the past. However, John should have addressed early on, Bridget's unplanned arrival to his office and explain that as a single father, spending long hours at work impacted his ability to spend quality time with his children. By validating his co-worker's presence and thanking her for coming by, John could have then provided the opportunity for an actually scheduled appointment to occur. The key here is maintaining open and honest communication, thereby alleviating the potential for assumptions to be made.

Males, just like females, can experience incivility and bullying within the workplace (Einarsen, 1999). John's victimization centered around his co-worker's perceptions of rejection, which in turn led to John being harassed by the co-worker and a staff nurse on his unit (Einarsen & Raknes, 1997). It is important that male nurses not dismiss false accusations made by male or female colleagues in the workplace. If bullying and incivility are suspected, steps should be taken to resolve the situation (refer to Chapter 4) immediately.

Resources for Nurses

1. **National Suicide Prevention Lifeline:** 1-800-273-8255

Website: https://suicidepreventionlifeline.org/

1. United Way 2-1-1- Provides information on available health and human services resources in the community (i.e. mental health services)

Website: https://www.211ct.org/

2. Occupational Safety and Health Administration (OSHA) - 1-800-321-6742 (OSHA)

Website: https://www.osha.gov/html/Feed_Back.html

3. **American Nurses Association:** 1-800-284-2378

Website: https://www.nursingworld.org/

Appendix 1 contains exploratory activities that discuss the impact of bullying and incivility on one's work-life and personal life. Self-esteem and self-worth are impacted by nurses who endure uncivil conduct in the workplace. The seeking of help in the workplace by nurses, is examined.

REFERENCES

Agency for Healthcare Research and Quality. (2019). *TeamSTEPPS*. Retrieved from https://www.ahrq.gov/teamstepps/index.html

Chen, C., Lin, C., Wang, S., & Hou, T. (2009). A study of job stress, stress coping strategies, and job satisfaction for nurses working in middle-level operating rooms. *The Journal of Nursing Research*, *17*(3), 199–210. doi:10.1097/JNR.0b013e3181b2557b PMID:19738448

Demerouti, E., Bakker, A. B., & Bulters, A. J. (2004). The loss spiral of work pressure, work-home interference and exhaustion: Reciprocal relations in a three-wave study. *Journal of Vocational Behavior*, *64*(1), 131–149. doi:10.1016/S0001-8791(03)00030-7

Demerouti, E., Bakker, A. B., Vardakou, I., & Kantas, A. (2003). The convergent validity of two burnout instruments: A multitrait-multimethod analysis. *European Journal of Psychological Assessment*, *18*, 296–307. doi:10.1027//1015-5759.19.1.12

Demerouti, E., & Nachreiner, F. (1998). The specificity of burnout in human services. Fact or artifact? *Zeitschrift fur Arbeitswissenschaft*, *52*, 82–89.

Einarsen, S. (1999). The nature and causes of bullying at work. *International Journal of Manpower*, *20*(1/2), 16–27. doi:10.1108/01437729910268588

Einarsen, S., & Raknes, B. I. (1997). Harrassment in the workplace and the victimization of men. *Violence and Victims*, *12*(3), 247–263. doi:10.1891/0886-6708.12.3.247 PMID:9477540

Huntington, A., Gilmour, J., Tuckett, A., Neville, S., Wilson, D., & Turner, C. (2011). Is anybody listening? A qualitative study of nurses' reflections on practice. *Journal of Clinical Nursing, 20*(9-10), 1413–1422. doi:10.1111/j.1365-2702.2010.03602.x PMID:21414055

Masalach, C. (1982). *Burnout: The cost of caring*. Englewood Cliffs, NJ: Prentice Hall.

Maslach, C., Jackson, S. E., & Leiter, M. P. (1996). Maslach Burnout Inventory Manual (3rd ed.). Palo Alto, CA: Consulting Psychologist Press.

Maslach, C., Schaufeli, W. B., & Leiter, M. P. (2001). Job burnout. *Annual Review of Psychology, 52*(1), 397–422. doi:10.1146/annurev.psych.52.1.397 PMID:11148311

Netemeyer, R. G., Boles, J. S., & McMurrian, R. (1996). Development and validation of work-family conflict—Work conflict scales. *The Journal of Applied Psychology, 81*(4), 400–410. doi:10.1037/0021-9010.81.4.400

Raja, U., Javed, Y., & Abbas, M. (2017, August 24). A time lagged study of burnout as a mediator in the relationship between workplace bullying and work-family conflict. *International Journal of Stress Management*. doi:10.1037tr0000080

Schmidt, B. J., MacWilliams, B. R., & Neal-Boylan, L. (2017). Becoming inclusive: A Code of conduct for inclusion and diversity. *Journal of Professional Nursing, 33*(2), 102–107. doi:10.1016/j.profnurs.2016.08.014 PMID:28363383

Weiland, D. (2015). Resilience to social bullying in academia: A phenomenological study. *Nurse Educator, 40*(6), 289–293. doi:10.1097/NNE.0000000000000169 PMID:25950796

APPENDIX 1

Exploration Activities

Directions: The purpose of the *Exploration Activities* are to encourage reflection on the issue of uncivil conduct in nursing by recording one's feelings about the act of incivility.

Why is the act of incivility so painful?

How has incivility effected your personal life?

How has incivility effected your work life?

Has incivility impacted your self-esteem?

Has incivility impacted your sense of self-worth?

Have you shared with a healthcare provider that you are experiencing bullying on your job? If no, why not? If yes, what did you share and what was the provider's response?

Do you feel that your complaints about the bully or bullies are being heard or understood at your job?

Do you feel that no one is interested in changing the bullying culture at your workplace?

____
____
____
____
____
____

Have you considered seeing a counselor or therapist?

____
____
____
____
____
____

If you do not feel you need to see a counselor or therapist to discuss the bullying you have experienced, what is your reason for making this decision?

____
____
____
____
____
____

Have you ever had thoughts of harming yourself or the bully (or bullies)? If yes, do you think that a counselor or therapist could help you resolve these feelings?---**It is important to seek help and resolve these feelings, harming yourself or another person is never the answer.**

____
____
____
____
____

Do you burden your family and friends with stories of the bullying that is occurring at work? And, do you think this is a healthy way to cope with the problem of the bullying?

Is it fair for your family and friends to have to carry the burden of fear, anxiety, and worry about you, when you can confide your emotional stress by forging a therapeutic relationship with a counselor or therapist?

Have you neglected your physical health problems that have developed as a result of the stress of the bullying experience (i.e. headaches and gastrointestinal problems)?

If you had the opportunity to resign your job tomorrow and move on to new employment, would you?

Do you feel that your current job is worth staying at, despite the uncivil behaviors of co-workers?

Do you feel empowered to address and bring resolution to the uncivil behaviors, and perpetrators of these acts, at your job?

If you left your job today, would you feel like you failed as a person, to protect yourself from self-harm or do you feel like you're leaving is solely for self-preservation?

Have you contemplated in therapy or counseling sessions, legal actions against the perpetrator?

Has therapy or counseling helped you make decisions that have had a positive impact on your ability to cope with incivility within the work environment?

How do you view yourself one year from now, with regard to the bullying situation?

Do you see yourself as being resilient?

Chapter 6
The Search for Support and Healing

ABSTRACT

Chapter 6 provides nurses, nurse leaders, and organizations interventions to understand, confront, and eliminate bullying and incivility from the workplace. Emotional intelligence (EI) and cognitive rehearsal are techniques when taught to nurses via in-services provided by organizations, can build awareness of verbal and nonverbal cues used in their communication as well as those of others. By understanding how we communicate and respond to others and vice versa, insight to what are appropriate and inappropriate responses can hold nurses accountable to how they treat one another. The neuroscience of oxytocin release at a biochemical level supports the benefits of organizations investing in the mental and physical health of their employees by empowering them to grow individually and as a collaborative team.

INTRODUCTION

Nurses affected by bullying in the workplace may ask themselves why they were targeted by the bully or bullies. This is a normal reaction. It is important for nurses to insightfully explore patterns of bullying sustained at more than one facility, and if this has been a repetitive issue for them during their career. Meeting with a counselor or therapist to discuss experienced patterns of bullying, can be beneficial to the victim. Blaming one's self for the negative behaviors of others, is not warranted and unproductive. Instead explore ways

DOI: 10.4018/978-1-5225-7341-8.ch006

of self-improvement and self-protection, so that bullying will be recognized and not tolerated in the future.

Asking Why You

Mental anguish over why one is being bullied will not end the bullying, nor help the nurse's immediate need for self-validation. If you are a nurse that is currently experiencing bullying, because of the risks for the development of health problems and depression and anxiety, it is imperative that help be sought immediately. The maintenance of one's mental and physical health should be the priority of the affected nurse. Additionally, affected nurses must ensure that the bullying is not compromising their own happiness within their personal life at home or with family and friends.

Never Isolate

When being bullied in the workplace, the tendency can be to isolate. Nurses working in toxic work environments may use silence and isolation as a means to self-protect. However, over time, this can impact them negatively within professional environments where collegiality and team work is emphasized. Ironically, as nurses attempt to use isolation to protect themselves, their work performance evaluations may identify their isolation as being suggestive of *lack of communication and not being a team player*.

Isolation for a brief period of time to gather one's thoughts and to regroup when a decline in work productivity secondary to workplace incivility has been identified, can be helpful. However, sustained patterns of isolation should be avoided. Nurses can self-protect in toxic work environments by disengaging from incivility during staff meetings and collaborations with negative peers. Nurses however, must maintain a physical presence and acknowledge their peers in a professional manner. Remember, while self- protection is paramount, the work of a nurse is what your health care facility or academic institution has hired you to do.

Organizational Strength

Health care organizations can help nurses experiencing bullying and incivility within the workplace by recognizing symptoms associated with dysfunctional microsystems (clinical units). Microsystems that have patterns of nurse turnover and reports from unions and Human Resources (HR) Departments of complaints of uncivil conduct; can be investigated monthly by administration. By holding managers and directors accountable monthly for reporting nurses resigning from their positions and reports to unions and HR, of unprofessional behaviors on the clinical unit, administration communicates a zero tolerance for workplace incivility.

Emotional Intelligence

Emotional intelligence (EI) is the ability of a person to recognize the emotions of others as well as their own. Nurses applying EI in their daily nursing practice, can differentiate between the emotional expressions of others in their work environment, and have insight into appropriate and inappropriate responses to others emotions. With this insight, nurses that are taught to apply EI in the workplace, can use it to guide their behavior and thinking in coping with incivility and bullying.

Nurses can effectively use EI to intervene and cope with incivility and bullying (Littlejohn, 2012; Salovey & Mayer, 1990; Meires, 2018) to protect themselves and other nurses in the workplace. Goleman (1997) views people as having two dimensions in the mind, the feeling mind and the thinking mind. Therefore, when nurses are taught to use their intellectual and rational thinking to understand why perpetrators react and respond, EI can be effective in nurses' decision as to how they will or will not respond to co-workers bullying and incivility behaviors and actions. EI can be used to regulate moods, control anger, and bring rational thinking to situations of uncivil conduct by nurses, so that perpetrators can be readily disempowered.

Health care organizations can implement workshops on the teaching of EI to promote workplace civility. Simulations are scenarios that are meant to emulate realistic situations. Workshops incorporating simulation scenarios to introduce the concept of EI and how it can be applied when nurses experience bullying and incivility in the workplace, can help nurses understand how to successfully deal with and resolve uncivil behaviors. According to Meires (2018), EI can be beneficial in the promotion of cultures of safety in health care environments. Particularly in the prevention of errors involving patient care, adverse events, the turnover of nursing staff, and low patient satisfaction scores (The Joint Commission, 2016).

Cognitive Rehearsal

Cognitive rehearsal is a technique that is used by therapist to assist clients/ patients in preparing for situations that they may encounter or have already encountered. With regard to bullying and incivility within the workplace, the technique of cognitive rehearsal can be taught to nurses, in the addressing uncivil conduct before it is encountered. Griffin and Clark (2014) recommend cognitive rehearsal as an intervention against lateral violence (displaced violence against one's peer) and incivility. Nurses can be taught within educational sessions provided by organizations, ways in which to practice how they would respond to a co-worker who is rude, engages with other perpetrators in mobbing behaviors and blames or attempts to belittle them.

Neuroscience and Organizational Health

Within social neuroscience, oxytocin is a hormone that is a neurochemical. Oxytocin (OT) plays a role in maternal-child bonding, social interaction, generosity, and empathy (Barraza & Zak, 2013). From a biochemical perspective when people work within organizational cultures that perpetuate either antisocial or trustworthiness, trustworthiness is associated with healthy work environments. Zak (2018) refers to these workplaces as high-trust organizations.

Hence, organizations that facilitate positive relationships, behaviors, and communication patterns among colleagues help their employees' brain synthesize oxytocin (Zak, 2018). Thereby, promoting employees' health. Zak (2018) identified eight essential factors that are necessary for organizations to build trust within their cultures. Zak uses the acronym OXYTOCIN. The eight factors are Ovation, eXpectation, Yield, Transfer, Openness, Caring, Invest, and Natural.

- **Ovation:** When organizations' recognize employees publically that perform their work well, OT is released. Organizations that develop a culture of publically recognizing employees' work performance have a decrease in staff turnover. According to Deloitte (2014), a global survey found that organizations that practice public recognition have 31% lower turnover of employees.

- **Expectation:** When employees decide to deal with challenges in the workplace as a group, OT is released. Team collaboration not only completes the work at hand in cooperation with others, but defeats isolation. With regard to workplace incivility and bullying, OT release can only occur when management sets a zero tolerance for uncivil conduct in the workplace. Zak (2018) stated, "Managers need to set hard but achievable *expectations* to stimulate colleagues' brains to synthesize OT" (p. 49).
- **Yield:** In organizations that support yield, employees decide how they will perform a task in absence of micromanagement. Leaders in high-trust organizations serve in the role of counselor and coach. Mistakes within *yield* organizations are viewed as opportunities for growth and learning. Collegiality and collaboration among employees as tasks are performed and projects completed, promote OT release (Zak, 2018).
- **Transfer:** Employees that exhibit *transfer* are able to demonstrate mastery and expertise at work in their specialty areas. Transfer can decrease employee stress of uncertainty and increase team motivation for the completion of projects (Zak, 2014). Employees have more autonomy because the organization appreciates their knowledge, therefore empowerment and self-efficacy levels are high. Hence, OT release is increased.
- **Openness:** When organizations' management and administration value transparency and *openness*, communication is candid, and trustworthiness among employees is high. With high trust worthiness, OT release will likely be high as well. It is important for organizations to maintain openness with their employees using all forms of technology (i.e. emails, intranet, etc.) as well as face-to-face communication within forums, grand rounds, and other types of meetings.
- **Caring:** The purpose of *caring* is to foster relationships among peers. The dynamics of relationships with colleagues within the work environment, when positive, can increase productivity. Because human beings by nature, are social, organizations where *caring* is promoted such as those having *bring your children to work days* or have on-site daycare, tend to have higher levels of OT in this area (Rath, 2006; Alexander & Zak, 2015).
- **Invest:** Organizations that *invest* monies and time into the training of their employees are more likely to have employees that are engaged. It is important that in conjunction with the training, employers provide

opportunities for their employees' personal growth and development (Ryff, 1995). The latter will increase OT.

- **Natural:** Within organizations whereby leadership is transparent, vulnerable and demonstrates integrity, these characteristics are more likely to be valued by their employees. These characteristics are *natural* and are conducive to the release of OT because the organization values trustworthiness (Aronson, Willerman, & Floyd, 1966).

Neurochemicals can affect one's psychological and physical health. For nurses experiencing bullying and incivility within the workplace, the stress that can occur with continual contact by perpetrators and negativity elicited by these interactions (or just being in the presence of the perpetrators), can inhibit OT. Hence, it is imperative that organizations that know that uncivil conduct is present in a work area(s), address the problem immediately.

By applying Zak's (2018) eight factors (OXYTOCIN) for the development of a high trust culture, organizations must first review each factor and determine if these supportive approaches exist or are absent in their work environments. Additionally, consider gathering data via a survey from employees, to assess if they feel safe in their workplace (i.e. absence of bullying, incivility and workplace violence), valued by their company, or are actively seeking employment elsewhere. Ensure that the survey is confidential and administered anonymously via a hyperlink. Organizations that develop a zero tolerance for uncivil behaviors, working collaboratively with their leadership, Human Resources, and their employees, can create healthier work environments.

Toolkits for Organizational Development

The purpose of these activities are to help organizational leadership inform, educate, and provide support to employees in the prevention of workplace bullying and incivility.

Case Study 10 is a hypothetical case study and all characters are fictional. In this case study, Wendy, a nurse on a clinical unit, encounters sarcastic comments about her hair.

Case Study 10: Wendy

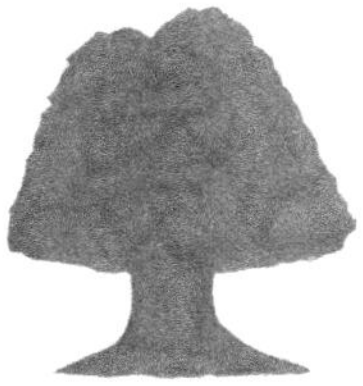

Wendy, a nurse on a medical unit, walks out of a patient's room after providing care. A nurse colleague, Belinda, makes a comment about Wendy's natural hair. Belinda states, "Wendy, do you really think an afro is appropriate for a professional setting? Maybe you should consider flat ironing your hair. It is so long and would look better straight." The comment was not in the context of being work-related, and caught Wendy off guard.

Wendy was always cordial in her interactions with Belinda. However, Belinda was at times very sarcastic and demeaning in her conversations with Wendy. Wendy is not certain how to deal with this situation, but she knows that something has to change. Belinda's negative interactions affect Wendy's workday. Wendy feels hurt and at times, perseverates on Belinda's negative statements and wonders if Belinda has any insight into her own behaviors.

Questions to Consider:

1. How would you advice Wendy on addressing Belinda's behaviors?

____
____
____
____
____

2. Do you think Belinda's comment about Wendy's natural hair is an EEOC violation?

____
____
____
____
____

3. Is Wendy being bullied?

____
____
____
____
____

Identify Weaknesses and Strengths

Nurses whom have experienced bullying can develop a distortion of self-concept. For example, the academically accomplished nurse may feel ill equipped to do the job for which he or she is well qualified to do and was hired for, because of the negative comments made by a bully (or bullies) regarding their qualifications, physical characteristics, or ability to perform the job. When nurses conduct a self-inventory of their skills, strengths, and weaknesses, they are able to determine their effectiveness in doing their job successfully with disregard to what the bully (or bullies) are attempting to do or say to discredit them.

It is helpful for nurses experiencing bullying to write an actual list of their strengths and weaknesses, while adding to the list work-life experiences, education, and specific training and qualifications to perform their job. This will help nurses affected by bullying to see for themselves, their own value and contributions to the workplace. Perceived weaknesses identified by perpetrators, may in fact be strengths that the bullied nurse was unaware that he or she had.

Nurses that experience bullying may repeat the bullies negative words to themselves via self-talk. This serves to undermine the nurse and creates low self-worth and low self-esteem. Nurses can learn to consciously reframe the negative self-talk by counteracting it with positive self-talk regarding their work-life accomplishments made, thereby disempowering the negative words of the bully.

Case Study 11 is a hypothetical case study and all characters are fictional. In this case study, Steve, a nurse on a Medical unit, encounters criticism from a co-worker, regarding his ability to interpret an electrocardiogram.

Case Study 11: Steve

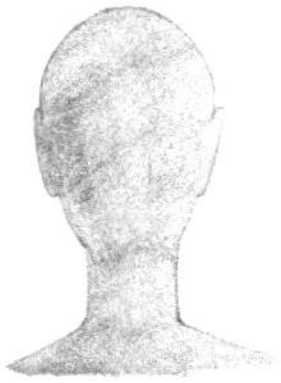

Marty and Steve are nurses on a Medical Unit that recently started admitting patients on telemetry. Marty and Steve received training in electrocardiogram (ECG) interpretation at the hospital. The two nurses had taken the class together just three months ago and both passed the course. However, Marty was constantly trying to correct Steve regarding his ability to interpret ECGs. Sometimes these verbal corrections occurred within patients' hospital rooms in front of the patients and family members. Steve was angry that Marty was publically humiliating him in front of his patients and their visitors. Steve wondered if he should address this issue with Marty directly or involve his nurse manager as a mediator to bring resolution to the situation.

Questions to Consider:

1. Have you ever felt humiliated in the workplace by someone challenging your knowledge on a topic or skill?

____

____

____

____

____

2. How did you resolve this issue?

____

____

____

____

____

3. Have you ever perseverated on comments made by other people? How did this make you feel?

____
____
____
____
____

4. Does Steve and Marty's situation constitute workplace bullying or incivility?

____
____
____
____
____

5. If you were Steve, how would you resolve this situation?

____
____
____
____
____

6. Is Marty a perpetrator of workplace incivility?

____
____
____
____
____

Case Study 12 is a hypothetical case study and all characters are fictional. In this case study, Cassandra, a nurse recalls being bullied at work. Cassandra is embittered by the situation and harbors anger directed at the perpetrator.

Case Study 12: Cassandra

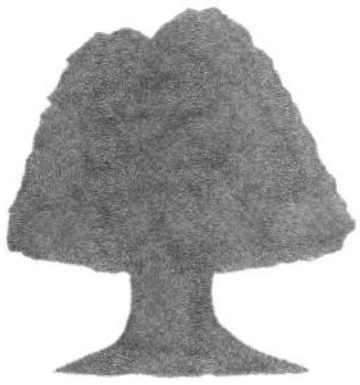

Cassandra during a lunch break at work with her colleague Sarah, shared that she was bullied at the hospital for seven years. Cassandra had recently accepted a position at a different hospital and after enduring the bullying in silence, now felt comfortable in sharing her experience. As she spoke about the incident and the perpetrator, every other word that proceeded out of her mouth included the statement, "I hate her."

Sarah listened in silence to Cassandra as she shared her bullying experience. Sarah noticed the more Cassandra used the words, "I hate her," her face became reddened in coloration and a scowl developed on her normally relaxed and beautiful face. Sarah watched as this calm and gentle woman she had known for several years, underwent a metamorphosis into an angry bitter human being.

Sarah found herself absorbing Cassandra' negative energy. Cassandra's emotional transformation was disturbing. One day when Cassandra and Sarah were once again having lunch together, Cassandra was angrily sharing past experiences she had with the perpetrator. Sarah reached across the table and lightly placed her right hand over Cassandra's left hand. Sarah's touching Cassandra's hand seemed to catch her off guard. Sarah asked for permission to take her pulse. The palms of her hands were warm and moist. Sarah took Cassandra's pulse for a full minute, it was 128 beats/per minute and slightly irregular. This was her resting heart rate.

Sarah shared with Cassandra her concern about her health. In response, Cassandra looked angrily at Sarah and said, "Don't worry about me. I am just fine." Cassandra abruptly ended the conversation and prepared to leave when Sarah asked, "What's his or her name?" Cassandra looked dumbfounded and asked, "Who?" Sarah paused, still sitting in a chair and stated, "The person you hate so much. The person who bullied you."

Cassandra began to cry. She shared, "Her name was Betty. She hurt me and made my life miserable." She sat back in her chair. Sarah spoke to Cassandra about the normalcy of hating Betty, but explained to her that her hatred of the perpetrator would only harm her. Cassandra disagreed with Sarah and abruptly left the hospital cafeteria. Sarah did not see Cassandra for about three months.

Hate Must End

After no contact, Cassandra called Sarah and asked to meet with her privately. Sarah invited Cassandra to come to her home for lunch. During lunch, Cassandra informed Sarah she had been diagnosed with new onset atrial fibrillation. Cassandra went on to explain that her cardiologist suggested that the atrial fibrillation was likely related to the stress she was under at work. She asked Sarah to help her with her hatred toward the person who bullied her.

Sarah listened to Cassandra as she shared her seven-year history of working with a nurse that bullied her. Sarah could not believe that she had endured this level of emotional abuse for seven years. It was then that Sarah understood why Cassandra used the word *hate* when she thought of her perpetrator.

Cassandra had been a devout Catholic for many years; Sarah asked to pray for Cassandra's health and healing (Seedall, Butler, & Elledge, 2014). In silence, the two colleagues held hands and prayed asking for healing from the anger Cassandra had towards Betty, the woman who had bullied her in the workplace. As they prayed, Cassandra held Sarah's hands tightly and as the prayer progressed; her grip loosened and was more relax.

Cassandra and Sarah agreed to meet for prayer at least once a week for 6-weeks. Their prayers focused on thanksgiving. By the fifth week, Cassandra's prayer was, "I am thankful that Betty entered my life, because I am a better person for it. I wish her well. And pray that whatever anger or hurt she has toward herself and others, is resolved." This was a complicated prayer given the bullying Cassandra sustained over time, but eventually her commitment to forgiveness ended the hate she held for her perpetrator. Prescribed Aspirin and Metoprolol to treat her atrial fibrillation, nine months later, Cassandra took only an aspirin. The atrial fibrillation resolved.

Lessons Learned

The emotion of hatred produces illness by mentally tormenting those who harbor it. When hatred is harbored for long periods of time, it can begin to attack the physical body. In Cassandra's case, her prolonged state of stress she experienced from bullying and the hatred she felt toward the perpetrator, likely led to the development of her cardiac illness (Harris, 2005; Toussaint, Williams, Musick, & Everson, 2001).

One could hypothesize that the intervention of the complimentary alternative therapy of prayer was beneficial to Cassandra in resolving her hatred. The intervention of prayer brought peace to Cassandra and reduced her stress, taking away her hatred toward her bully. Thus, prayer was a positive intervention that had the long-term effect of healing a physical problem.

Ultimately, the forgiveness (Enright & Fitzgibbons, 2015) and thanksgiving components of prayers over the 6-week time period, were beneficial in helping Cassandra start a new journey in her life. Cassandra can now begin her new job and live her life without a cardiac dysrhythmia. Most importantly, she released herself from the emotional bondage that her bully Betty had over her for so many years.

The Amygdala

The amygdala consists of two almond shaped nuclei clusters within the central nervous system. Situated near the front of the temporal lobe of the two cerebral hemispheres, the amygdala is part of the limbic system. With stimulation of the amygdala, humans can experience the following: temporary amnesia, confusion, disturbed awareness, and fear (McCance & Heuther, 2018).

The amygdala is involved in the fight-or-flight response. Glutamate is one of the neurotransmitters released within the brain that can cause persons to become excitable. During the fight-or-flight response, the adrenal glands produce adrenaline and cortisol in response to stress and fear.

Theoretically, with workplace incivility being experienced by a nurse on a routine basis, the body could eventually enter states of fight-or-flight because of prolonged periods of stress and fear. Cassandra's diagnosis of a new onset atrial fibrillation could have occurred as a result of the seven years of intermittent bullying in the workplace that she was exposed to. With workplace bullying, it is not known by the victim when the next attack will be orchestrated. Thereby causing the victim of bullying to maintain a nearly constant state of fear.

Do Not Blame Yourself

Avoid blaming yourself for the behaviors of the bully directed toward you. Recognize that the perpetrator of bullying is subject to free will, and has a right to make any decision that they deem correct. But, so does the nurse affected by bullying. The nurse affected by bullying has the right to protect themselves and defend their right to act professionally within a professional environment. This means, having the right not to condone uncivil behaviors in the workplace perpetrated against oneself.

Berndsen, Wenzel, Thomas, and Noske (2017) noted that nurses whom are bullied in the workplace may exhibit perceived perspective-taking. Perceived perspective-taking occurs when the nurse affected by bullying perceives that the perpetrator is sensitive and feels moral emotions. By demonstrating empathy towards the perpetrator, the affected nurse becomes more conciliatory. This emotional response by the affected nurse, can aid in the reconciliation process by helping the affected nurse to forgive the perpetrator.

Forgiveness can bring healing to victims (Enright & Fitzgibbons, 2015). Hate is a volatile emotion that can be detrimental to the overall health of victims of bullying. When someone that has been bullied makes the conscious decision to forgive their perpetrator, this does not mean that they are opening themselves up to be abused again. Forgiveness should not be equated to acceptance of harm or injury by another person, but releasing one's self from emotional pain experienced by the bully (or bullies). Thereby, disempowering the bully (or bullies).

Get the Help You Need

Van Vliet (2008) applied grounded theory methodology in a study exploring the experience of shame and resilience. Participants in the study were 13 adults that were interviewed by Van Vliet and audiotaped during face-to-face interviews. Results indicated that participants conceptualized shame as being an assault on themselves, whereby the sense of power and control, self-concept, and social connection is violated. Hence, there is an attack on one's self.

In applying Van Vliet's study to bullying, nurses affected by workplace bullying may feel inadequate because they may not initially be able to protect themselves from the negative attacks of the perpetrator(s). Or, the affected nurse may wonder why they may not have been readily able to identify the perpetrator's behaviors as incivility. Regardless of the origin of the shame, it is important for nurses affected by bullying to forgive themselves, so that self-care can be initiated and emotional healing from the bullying experience can begin.

Be Open to the Assistance of Others

The nurse that is experiencing bullying may isolate themselves in the workplace in an attempt to avoid trusting others. This avoidance of others is self-protective, but can be detrimental because the nurse may potentially lose the support of peers within the organization. These peers can provide support to the nurse as he or she deals with the emotional and physical complexities of incivility. According to Zak (2018), "Human beings are embedded in various organizations. Organizational cultures can promote prosocial behaviors such as trustworthiness or antisocial behaviors such as theft" (p. 45). Healthy organizations promote trustworthiness and employees are more likely to feel safe in these workplaces.

It is important for nurses to adapt models of motivation and theories of self-determination, as they make the conscious decision to no longer permit bullying in the workplace. When nurses learn to successfully navigate the health care (or academic) system, in order to resolve uncivil conduct, they are empowered to reorder their lives and rid themselves of the incivility they experienced. Healthy relationships both within the work environment and in one's personal life, can be beneficial in aiding the nurse in the seeking of an existence in absence of the bullying perpetrator(s).

Forgiveness

When nurses impacted by bullying forgive the perpetrator(s), their own victimhood ends and they feel empowered to progress despite the actions of the perpetrator(s). Forgiveness disables punishment (Strelan, 2017). Although affected nurses may contemplate retribution against the perpetrator(s), forgiveness releases the nurses emotionally, to heal.

Questions to Consider

1. How does forgiving the perpetrator(s) help me?

2. Do you feel any connectedness to the person who bullied you?

____
____
____
____
____
____
____

3. I know I have to forgive my bully or I could potentially harbor hate that can be just as emotionally crippling as the bullying behaviors themselves. I can forgive this person (or persons) by:

____
____
____
____
____
____
____

Case Study 13 is a hypothetical case study and all characters are fictional. In this case study, Michael, a nurse that experienced bullying in the workplace, reflects on how the experience affected him.

Case Study 13: Michael

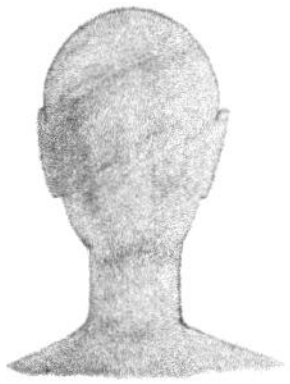

A nurse bullied Michael on his unit for one year. Michael, because of the workplace bullying he experienced, disengaged from his relationships with other colleagues on the unit. Michael was unaware he did this, but was in self-protective mode.

After the bullying ended, Michael began to reengage with his colleagues because he felt more relaxed in the workplace environment. He received support from those colleagues that were aware of the bullying he had endured. Michael began to feel valued by peers and his self-confidence increased. Michael shares, "I see myself as a strong person that was misled by the negative opinions of others and rescued by my decision to resiliently survive workplace bullying."

Questions to Consider

1. Can maintenance of positive peer relationships within the workplace and in one's personal life, benefit the nurse that is being bullied?

____

____

____

____

____

____

2. Can nurses affected by bullying, make the conscious decision to eventually reconcile with their perpetrator(s)?

____

____

____

____

____

____

TOOLKITS FOR NURSES

The Toolkit of Mindfulness: Self-Care

Mindfulness mediation is a form of mental retraining of the human brain. The practice of mindful meditation has no association with a religion, and therefore can be practiced by agnostics, atheists, and persons with a religious affiliation. Mindfulness is comprised of different types of meditation such as breathing exercises, mindful eating, mindful listening, and mindful mental exercises with the focus of the removal of negative thought processes. Negative thought processes cause one to worry, perseverate and become anxious. Persons who practice mindful meditation learn to recognize the origin of negative thoughts without empowering these thoughts to linger within the conscious mind. Victims of incivility therefore learn to immediately release the negative thoughts and replace them with positive more empowering words. Mindfulness teaches the victim of incivility to be kind and compassionate with themselves.

Nurses enter a profession that cares for others. Mindfulness meditation, teaches nurses to care for themselves while being in-tuned to the needs of others. Nurses practicing mindfulness learn to be in-tuned to their environments by applying all of the senses (i.e. sight, touch, smell, taste, and hearing), and examining how their interaction with the environment impacts them. For example, listening intently to others, appreciating the taste of a food item and its texture in the mouth as the food is swallowed, helps nurses to mentally slow their thinking and relax. Smelling a flower and touching its delicate petals helps the mindful nurse appreciate beauty in simplicity.

By learning to appreciate each day and making the familiar new, forgiving others and one's self, paying attention to one's environments, awakening the senses, and relaxing one's breathing (Mayo Clinic, 2015), nurses can gradually decrease their stress. While mindfulness may not work for everyone, it introduces relaxation techniques that can be practiced in ways that may feel safer to nurses based upon their comfort level. For example, learning to slow breathing down could be done as the nurse listens to music or takes a walk outside. Meditation can be completed not by using a mindfulness exercise such as the observance of a flower or other object, but by praying or repeating a scripture for spiritual support.

Regardless of how nurses decide to apply mindfulness exercises to stress reduction, self-care is paramount. In this chapter mindful exercises will be used to help nurses apply basic self-care techniques before the work day begins, during the work day, and at the end of the work day. Practice these techniques at least 15 to 20 minutes daily for approximately 8 to 9 weeks.

Case Study 14 is a hypothetical case study and all characters are fictional. In this case study, Margaret is a nurse that bullies others in the workplace.

Case Study 13: Margaret

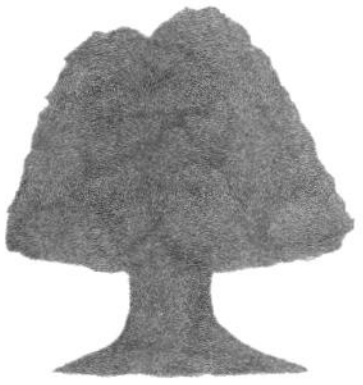

Margaret has been an oncology nurse for 32 years. In her care of patients, she is kind and exhibits compassion. However, in her interactions with nursing colleagues, she is argumentative, ends conversations abruptly, and demeaning of the skills and knowledge level of other nurses. Margaret has had multiple complaints by co-workers of bullying, all of which she has successfully disputed. The healthcare organization's response to the management of Margaret's behaviors, has been to relocate her to one of the three specialty oncology units within the hospital system.

Margaret was diagnosed with breast cancer eight months ago. She has received chemotherapy and is now receiving radiation therapy. After a six-month leave for treatment of her cancer, Margaret returned to work. In her absence from the clinical unit, a new graduate nurse, Rebecca was hired. Rebecca is highly motivated and quickly retains new knowledge. The climate of the oncology unit has changed in Margaret's absence. Nursing staff are more supportive of one another. Rebecca, in collaboration with other nurses on the unit, has instituted *staff nights out*. During the *staff nights out*, nursing staff meet at a restaurant to relax, chat, and eat together.

The unit manager, Rebecca, and other nursing staff welcome Margaret back with a celebratory luncheon and Margaret is given a gift from the staff. Margaret completed her radiation therapy and her health is improving. Four months status post the completion of cancer treatment, Margaret's interactions on the unit with fellow nurse colleagues have become volatile. Targeting Rebecca, she has been observed by other staff making negative comments during situation, background, assessment and recommendation (SBAR) report handoffs. Margaret insults Rebecca and challenges her ability to care for complex cancer patients. Rebecca, whom is normally a happy, engaged and highly productive nurse, is becoming withdrawn.

Rebecca's colleagues noticing the change in her behavior, discuss their concerns with her. Rebecca tearfully shares how Margaret has been making rude remarks and demeaning of her abilities as a nurse. Rebecca empowered by her colleagues, completes a detailed chronological document outlining the situations in which dialogues with Margaret were uncivil. The document is shared with the nurse manager and Human Resources.

Rebecca meets with the nurse manager and a Human Resources representative and a documented formal complaint is completed and placed within Margaret's employee record. Margaret is placed on progressive disciplinary action. However, the bullying persists.

One weekend, when Rebecca is on the unit documenting late after an emergent code involving a patient that had a cardiac arrest, Margaret berates her about not administering a medication to a patient that was due at the time that the code was occurring. Rebecca begins to cry uncontrollably as the berating persists, even as Rebecca attempts to walk away from the situation, Margaret follows her. A co-worker notifies the nursing supervisor who arrives on the clinical unit accompanied by a hospital security officer. The nursing supervisor tries to calm Margaret down, but to no avail; she is asked to pack up her belongings and leave hospital grounds.

After an investigation of the incident, Margaret is terminated. Her service to the hospital as a registered nurse for 32 years is ended. However, the destructiveness of her incivility remains as Rebecca begins the healing process as a victim of incivility.

Mindful Healing

A fellow nurse introduces mindfulness to Rebecca. Rebecca learns to recognize how the negative interactions she mentally recalls having with Margaret, cause her to feel insecure and inadequate. Applying mindfulness techniques, Rebecca is able to recognize these interactions as being merely words facilitating an emotional response. Williams and Penman (2012) describe emotions as bundles of feelings, thoughts, impulses, and bodily sensations. These emotional bundles can be regulated and controlled when mindfulness is used to bring awareness to the victim of incivility, that the negative thoughts recalled, have no power unless perseverated upon. Meditation and breathing exercises can be used to stop the process of engaging negative thoughts and bring focus to the value of calmness, an appreciation and recognition of one's surroundings, and a soothing of the troubled mind.

SIMPLIFYING AND APPRECIATING: NURSES' APPLICATION OF MINDFUL EXERCISES

Mindfulness Exercise: Toothbrush Meditation

Step 1: Becoming Aware

Each day you use an item that helps make your day easier, or may help you facilitate self-care for yourself or others. In this meditation you will be focusing on the use of a toothbrush. As you stand at your bathroom sink, ensure that you are standing in front of a mirror.

- Look at the toothbrush. Examine its bristles. Are the bristles worn and bent showing overuse? Or are the bristles upright and clean?
- Examine the head of the toothbrush. Are there bite marks from your teeth? How does the remainder of the toothbrush look and feel?
- Place toothpaste on the toothbrush. Watch the toothpaste as you slowly place it on the brush. Now, place the toothbrush in your mouth. Taste the flavor of the toothpaste as you gently begin massaging in a circular motion, your gums and teeth. What sensations are you feeling right now?

Figure 1. Toothbrush meditation

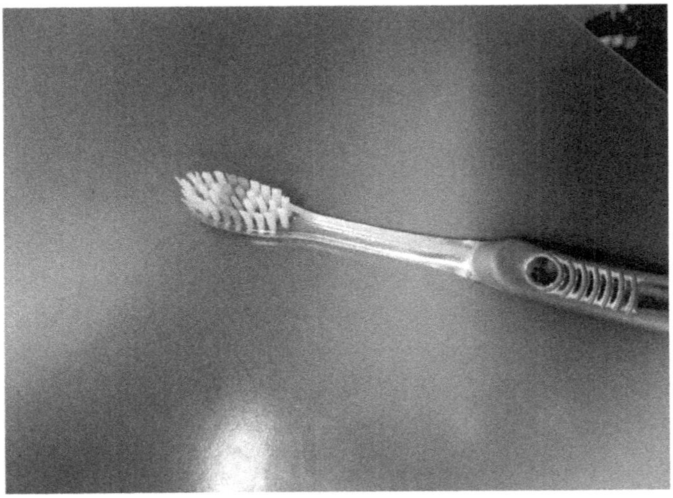

Step 2: Gathering and Focusing Attention

Redirect your attention to the purpose of brushing your teeth. Mouth hygiene is important in preservation of health because it prevents dental caries and reduces bacterial growth in the mouth. You are brushing your teeth because you care about your appearance, oral hygiene, and health.

Step 3: Expanding Attention

Notice how you are standing in front of the sink and mirror in the bathroom. Is your posture slumped over? Are you standing upright? If you are slumping, stand tall with your shoulders back. Proudly brush your teeth. Self-care is important, you are important.

Step 4: Wash Away the Unclean

Rinse your mouth out using a cup of water. Swish the water in your mouth and expectorate. Examine your teeth and gums. Your mouth should feel cleaner. You should feel proud because you took the time to care for yourself. Assess your mouth to determine whether there are particles or traces of food left in the mouth. Floss between your teeth, and rinse again.

MINDFULNESS EXERCISE

Mindfulness Exercise: Smile Meditation

Step 1: Becoming Aware

Each day represents a new day and new start. The smile meditation is meant to help you embrace the start of a new day and be thankful that you are glad to have awaken from sleep to be a part of this day. This meditation begins with you lying in bed. Smile, as you close your eyes and deeply inhale. Count to three slowly 1…2… and… 3. Breathe out slowly to the count of 1…2… and…3.

Figure 2. Smile meditation

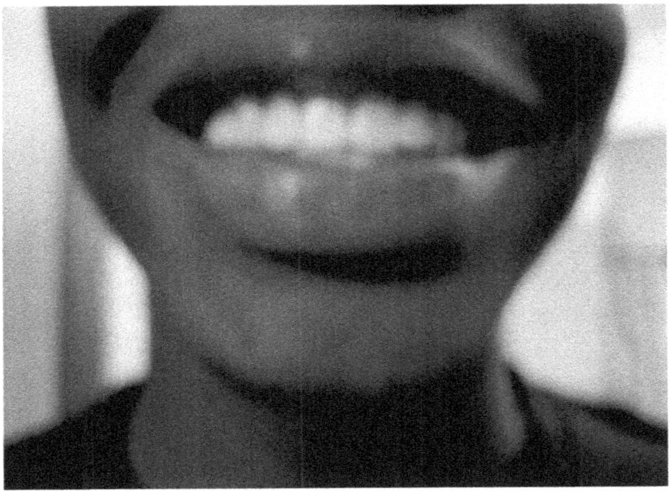

Step 2: Gathering and Focusing Attention

Smile as you open your eyes and scan the room. Arise from your bed and still smiling, lift your arms up high as if you are touching the ceiling and stretch. Smile and relax your body as the stretch ends.

Step 3: Expanding Attention

Take a slow walk around your home and smile as you notice and see things and people that you are thankful for. As you see a family member, smile and acknowledge their presence with a hug. Tell that person that you are thankful for them being in your life. After walking around your home, smile again and begin your day.

MINDFUL EXERCISE

Mindfulness Exercise: Breathe out Stress and Breathe in Peace

This exercise can be performed during a 15-minute break at work. Find a quiet area. Sit down in a chair with your shoulders back and posture straight in the chair. Close your eyes and visualize a light blue sky on a clear, warm day. Breathe out the stress……Breathe in peace. Count 1, 2, 3, 4, and 5. Repeat at least 4 times.

Nurses Toolkit for Self-Care: Exercise

Stress Reduction Walk at Work

During a 15-minute break, when possible, leave the unit and take a walk outside circling the facility at least once. If the weather is inclement, take the steps in a stairwell within the facility. When you take the time to add exercise to a busy day, you are providing self-care and have given yourself time away

Figure 3. Breathe out stress and breathe in peace

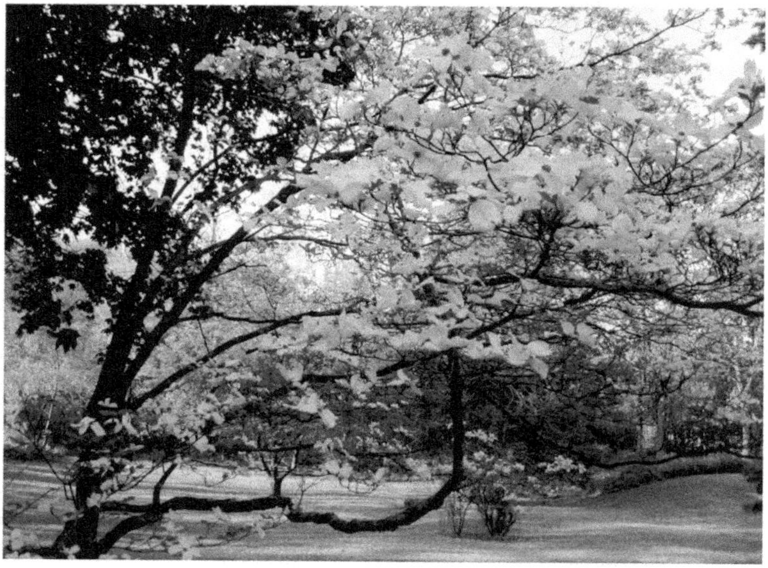

Figure 4.

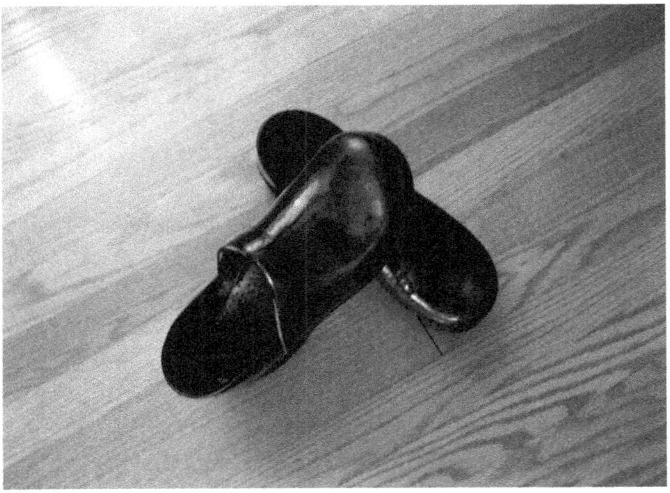

from the business of work and related stress. Drink water before and after you walk to maintain hydration. Once you feel comfortable with your stress reduction walks, you can gradually increase the pace.

Toolkit for Nurses: Hydrate and Eat Healthy

Hydrate and Eat Healthy

It is important to eat healthy and hydrate. Ensure that you diet includes lean meats, fish, a carbohydrate (i.e. brown rice or sweet potato), vegetables and fruit. Hydrate with water throughout the day. Snacks can include a low sodium and low sugar protein bar or a plain yogurt with added nuts, grains, and fruit for flavoring. A healthy diet can enhance energy and vitality for a body and mind under stress from toxic work environments.

Write down a healthy lunch or dinner that you can bring to work to eat.

____

____

____

____

Figure 5.

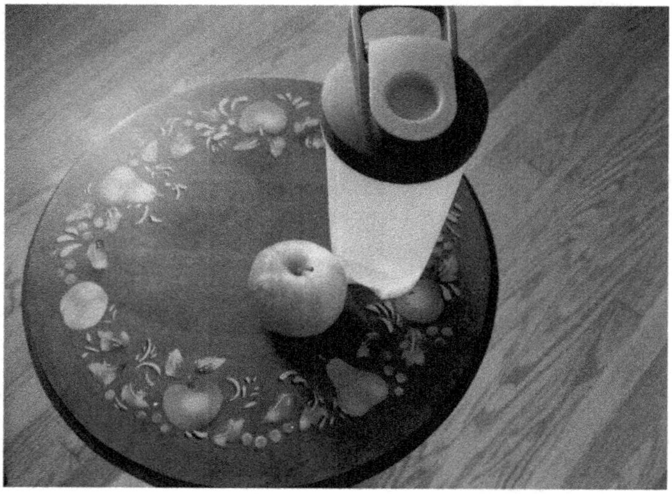

Write a healthy snack and beverage that you can bring to work.

___

___

___

Toolkit for Nurses: Self-Care Is Important

Self-care regimens should include healthy eating, hydrating with water, and exercise in order to maintain optimal function and health. Bullying is psychologically and physically damaging to victims. The materialization of constant falsehoods and accusations, often not known by the victim, but facilitated by the perpetrator(s), can make the victim feel paranoid. Sleeplessness, poor appetite, and constant perseveration on the episodes of bullying, can prove overwhelming to the victim, thereby impacting their health.

Valuing one's self is taking the time to care for one's physical, spiritual, and emotional needs. Workplace incivility can drain affected nurses of their ability to care for themselves. The covert and overt displays of incivility by perpetrators, can be frustrating and overwhelming for affected nurses (Dzurec, Kennison, and Albataineh, 2014).

Nurses are encouraged to report bullying as soon as possible. By seeking assistance from supervisors, employee assistance programs, human resources, and when applicable, unions, and employment attorneys; substantial mental and physical damage incurred by affected nurses (Rodwell & Demir, 2012; Wieland & Beitz, 2015) can be avoided. Practicing self-care, while seeking an end to the bullying and workplace incivility, not only empowers affected nurses, but may promote health and wellness.

TOOLKIT FOR NURSES: MEDITATIONS

Meditations

Directions: Find a quiet area. These meditations were developed to help you reclaim your identity, self-esteem, and self-worth that existed before you experienced workplace incivility and bullying. Use these meditations to empower yourself and take away the presumed power of the bully or bullies within your workplace.

Figure 6. Woman Untitled

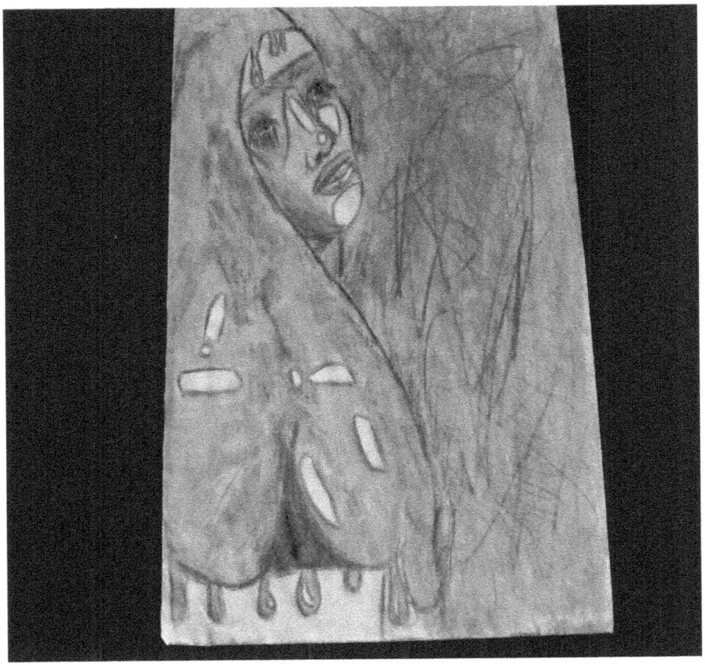

Meditation One: Worry Release

Being bullied can cause a person to feel devalued. You may be worrying about what others think about you. Examples of thoughts could be:

"Am I smart enough?"

"Did I do a good job today at work?"

"What could I have done to make others not like me?"

"How do I try to fit in?"

Release your worries. These are only words playing in your head like a tape recorder. Cut off the tape and set it to erase. Instead, ask these questions of your bully or bullies-

"Who are you to think that with all I have accomplished before meeting you, that you can define me?"

"Are you so insecure that you feel threatened by my very existence?"

"I am smart and very capable of doing my job"

"I love who I am and you have no power over me."

Releasing the worry empowers the nurse affected by bullying to recognize and value his or her own gifts.

Meditation Two: Forgiveness

The unnecessary pain evoked by someone who does not know me well. A pain unprovoked, arising from your (the perpetrator's) own insecurities. I have no shame, for I have not forfeited my dignity on your (the perpetrator's) behalf, nor will I. I forgive you (the perpetrator) because I have made the conscious decision to not allow your (the perpetrator) negativity to have any significance in my life. I have moved on.

Meditation Three: Decision

Conscious decisions of disempowerment. Quiet is the mind that pays no attention to intentional incivility. A decision has been made. Closure to negativity and openness to the positivity that envelopes my mind. A conscious decision has been made and you (the perpetrator) have no power.

Meditation Four: Shhhhh Silence

Guide your mind to listen to silence. The busyness of the day ends when silence is embraced. Say aloud *shhhh* and consider its meaning. A finger placed over pursed lips. A reminder that a disturbance is not desired.

Meditation Five: The Value of Self

I am invaluable. Priceless, more than rare metals or jewels. I have a name__________________ (say your own name in full--- first, middle, and last name). I existed before (say the perpetrator(s) name(s) entered my life and I will exist after this bullying ends.

Repeat this meditation at least three times a day; before work, during work, and at the end of work. Your home life is your sanctuary. Maintain a work-life balance by avoiding bringing your workplace issues home, whenever possible.

Meditation Six: Facing Perpetrators

Violence against a perpetrator is never an answer. It is important that victims of bullying never resort to harming anyone. This meditation allows you to stroll by your perpetrators in the workplace, unafraid and unintimidated.

Walk upright and strong as you walk in the hallways at work. Be aware of your posture. You appear professional and polished. No one is like you at your workplace. The mold truly has been broken. As you walk pass the bully or bullies, make eye contact and pass by them unafraid. Your walk is easy, unrushed and a stroll in appearance. You have nothing to be afraid of.

Go about your day and do the work well, that you were hired to perform. You are capable and can easily make eye contact with the bully and be unfazed by their presence. Stroll by, make eye contact, do your job, and enjoy your day.

Repeat These Words: I walk boldly. I know who I am.

Meditation Seven: In the Here and Embracing the Now

Sometimes it can be difficult to see past the pain of the day, especially when you are being bullied. Learning to embrace the here and now is important because it puts perspective on situations. The longevity of a day will end within 24-hours and that day will never again exist. Never give a day that can never be lived again in your lifetime, to a bully (or bullies).

Repeat These Words: This is a new day. I can breathe in the newness of this day and all the positive expectations that I can help make happen. I do not have to seek for, nor embrace the negative. I embrace the here and now because I am blessed to be alive within this day, and I choose to let no one dictate how I feel within this day. I embrace the here and now fully!

Meditation Eight: Pathways to Tranquility

Take a walk today. Before you go for a walk, map out your path in your head. Imagine the steps you will take and what you will see if the pathway is familiar to you. Prepare for your walk. Be mindful of how you are preparing. Put on comfortable clothing and shoes. If your walk will be long, bring a bottle of water.

Open your door and begin your path. Examine the world around you. Is it a busy city street with sounds of horns, a school bus passing by, and people talking on their phones? Or is it a quiet suburb, with the occasional sound of a closing car door as people depart for the start of their day or someone jogging or walking pass you?

No matter where you are, seek and listen for birds, look for green grass, or a plant within or around your pathway. Examine the ground for rocks, pavers, sidewalks, soil, and sand. Feel and listen to the changes in levels of the pathway as you move toward your desired destiny.

Pathways, organized and unplanned, can be made tranquil by you. The decision to alter your path is not the decision of others, but is your decision. Noise may be present in your pathway, but you can choose to filter what you hear and focus on all things beautiful and calm and peaceful in your path.

Listen to your breathing and your steps as you determine your path. Regulate your pace. Speed up your pace, then slow it down. This is your pathway and tranquility belongs to you alone.

Meditation Nine: Leaping Over Negativity

There are times when you will feel that obstacles are in your way. Be it at work, home, or other settings, thoughts of defeat may envelope you. Consider, what is my obstacle? What have I allowed to get in the way of embracing positivity, of being happy, and of being healthy?

Write down on a small piece of paper, an obstacle in your way. If it is a person write their name on the piece of paper. If it is yourself, write your own name on the paper. Perhaps you have a financial obstacle or an emotional or spiritual burden, write these also on a separate piece of paper.

Take these pieces of paper with you to an open space that is quiet and scatter these pieces of paper around the floor. Look at each piece of paper, and say the name of the obstacle aloud. Then, leap over the obstacle because you have already defeated it. Repeat this process until you have successfully leaped over every obstacle you have written on a piece of paper.

Gather each piece of paper, read the names of the obstacles aloud again and say these words, "Obstacles, you are defeated and have no power over me." Throw your obstacles away in the trash. Move forward today, with the visualization that you have leaped over your negativity and have control over how you perceive and interact with your obstacles that exist in your life.

TOOLKITS FOR NURSES: OTHER SELF-CARE TECHNIQUES

What Is Reiki?

Reiki is a complimentary alterative therapy that is energy-based. Originally developed in Japan, the Reiki practitioner uses the palms of their hands to transfer energy to their clients. This transferred energy can promote physical and emotional healing. Reiki can be beneficial to nurses that have been bullied in helping them release negative emotions and facilitate healing.

Therapeutic Massage

Therapeutic massage can help reduce pain, relax tense muscles, improve circulation, and decrease stress. Nurses affected by workplace bullying may benefit from a massage. Therapeutic massages can help reduce stress. Nurses can purchase a service plan with a massage therapist to receive one massage a month as a means to reduce their stress and decrease their use of the service plan to as needed, once stress decreases.

Positive Affirmations

Directions: Positive affirmations are words or statements to help improve one's perceptions of themselves. These words or statements are self-empowering, positive and foster a healthy mental attitude. Read each positive affirmation and fill in the blanks addressing your specific situation.

Positive Affirmation One: I Have Won This Battle

I have won this battle________________________________. I am not alone in this situation. I can call upon____________________________ for help. I was hurt by____________________________, but this hurt has ended. I will not gi ve____________________________ or any other person(s), control over me. My life and destiny do not belong to ____________________________. I am greater than the words and actions of ________________________ ____________. I have already won this battle. You________________ _______________ need only to wave your white flag as I walk past you ________________________. Greatness awaits me and overcomes all the doubt. I walk in solitude, peace, and with grace. I have won this battle.

Positive Affirmation Two: Loneliness

Loneliness is not my name. Heartache is not a pathway I have to take. Watch your words________________________________. The negativity and hatred do not belong to me. Critical words said, skepticism, and cynical, I move forward beyond your own insecurities____________________________. Your words define your insecurities, not mine. I smile. Your attempts to impose your own loneliness upon me have failed. I wish you well and move forward. Loneliness is not my name. My name is________________________.

Positive Affirmation Three: Tears

My name is____. You can only call me______________________________________. I will not cry any more tears over your bitter words directed unprovoked, toward me. I am strong, capable, beautiful, and kind. I am greater than any negative words that you can verbalize.

Positive Affirmation Four: Home

My home is my sanctuary. Your name (the perpetrator(s)) has been spoken in my home, a distraction from my peace within my sanctuary. My family comes first and home is a place of laughter and rebirth of spirit. Your (the perpetrator(s)) negativity is not welcomed in my home. I have decided that peace for me is a priority and peace in my home with my family is important! Home is my___________________________ and I will not give to you (the perpetrator(s)) the honor of speaking your (the perpetrator(s)) name.

Positive Affirmation Five: Overcomer

Openness to the new. A day ended and your presence less prominent. Frustration ended, health restored, and kinder times envelop me. Overcomer of the nonsensical words spoken by___________________________.

Positive Affirmation Six: Forgiveness

I choose to forgive____ (the perpetrator's name(s)). While I do not understand the pain that _______________________________ (the perpetrator's name(s)) has gone through that has caused them to be bitter and exhibit negative behaviors that harm others, it is my hope that they one day seek help to resolve their problems. I will no longer own someone else's hatred, anger, and frustration. I choose to forgive. I choose to have peace in my life.

TOOLKIT FOR NURSES: EMPOWERMENT

Ending Bullying Starts With Me

Discussions about how bullying can be ended were made in previous chapters of this book. However, emphasis must be placed on the importance of nurses taking responsibility for their professional conduct in the workplace. Nurses are obligated to protect and care for patients. The care of patients is a priority that far outweighs any issues of conduct among health care professionals. It is imperative that nurses work collaboratively with managers, human resources, and administration in holding bullies accountable for workplace disruptions. Nurses can accomplish this, by upholding the American Nurses Association's Code of Ethics that supports a zero tolerance for non-inclusive behaviors. Protect your patients, protect yourself, protect your license, and protect your fellow nurses.

An Unnecessary Grief

Incivility is an *unnecessary grief.* An unnecessary grief is a disruption in one's life that has no benefit, nor provides support or healing, only a period of mourning within one's spirit. When a spirit is in mourning, it theoretically, grieves what use to be. For the nurse that is being bullied, what use to be or formally exist, was peace in absence of bullying and incivility.

The period of time, no matter how long or short that a nurse endures bullying, can strip the nurse of their confidence, ability to concentrate, and overall self-concept. While the nurse remains cognizant of the reality that the bully or bullies in the workplace, do not have ultimate control over their life, the intrusive thoughts and moments of negative encounters with bullying bombard the affected nurse's thoughts. An *unnecessary grief* develops as the nurse enters a period of frustration, disbelief, and shock of how the negative behaviors of others has impacted their personal and professional life.

Overcoming the experience of bullying as an *unnecessary grief* can be done. The solution is to begin approaching each day at work as one that will be absent of all bullying experiences. This means not acknowledging bullying behaviors. The nurse must arrive at work with a predetermined plan of how the day's work will be completed. While the plan may vary based upon unforeseen circumstances, having distinct time frames to complete different work-related tasks, can allow the nurse to minimize the potential encounters with the bully.

All encounters with the bully or bullies should be treated as inconveniences in one's predetermined work plan. The affected nurse must realize, in actuality, the bully or bullies are nuisances that disrupt productivity. When affected nurses are able to conceptualize bullying this way, it will eventually seem incomprehensible why these often emotionally damaged men and women, were permitted to have power over the affected nurses in the first place.

The workplace is a means for nurses to obtain and establish an income. In absence of work, bills cannot be paid, food cannot be purchased, and shelter cannot be sustained. Bullies, tolerated in the workplace, can lead to affected nurses resigning from jobs that they enjoy and that financially meet the needs of themselves and their family members. It is for that reason, that nurses must eventually reach the conclusion, that bullies are merely an *unnecessary grief*, and the perceived power over their victims can be nullified by not acknowledging their acts and dismissing insecure attacks on other nurses they work with, in order to validate their existence and own abilities in the workplace.

Seeking Recourse to Protect Others

Bullying is seldom done in isolation. Once a bully knows that they can get away with harassing one person, they will inevitably, attempt to do it to others. This behavior is likely linked to the need for the bully to exert power over others because they themselves feel powerless. Therefore, if a nurse is experiencing bullying in the workplace, it may behoove the nurse to investigate patterns of bullying existing with other co-workers by the same perpetrator.

By investigating patterns of bullying, the nurse validates that the source of the problem is likely not them, but based on the bully's thwarted view of reality. It is important that nurses affected by bullying collaboratively work together to end it. Nurses can help maintain healthy and safe work environments by documenting and reporting uncivil behaviors.

Reports of uncivil behaviors can be made by nurses to their manager and human resources in writing and verbally in face-to face meetings. Uncivil conduct is not conducive to the workplace and impacts nurses' ability to care for themselves, patients, and their families because of the mental distress they experience secondary to bullying. Seeking ways to protect themselves and others, can help nurses begin the healing process and empower them to end incivility within their work environments.

Progression Beyond the Pain

Nurses impacted by bullying experience physical symptoms that have effected a body consumed with worry, anger, frustration, and distrust. Physiological symptoms may emerge as nontraditional stress symptoms or vague complaints. Nurses, although skilled in the assessment of health ailments, may be unable to make the direct connection of their declining health to being bullied. The following are signs and symptoms that nurses may experience that are likely related to their being bullied:

Signs and Symptoms Associated With Bullying

- Weight loss
- Neck Pain
- Back Pain
- Jaw Pain (Grinding of Teeth)
- Nail Biting
- Nausea and Vomiting
- Tension Headaches
- Indigestion
- Sleeplessness
- Fatigue
- Generalized Bodily Aches
- Poor Appetite
- Hair Loss
- Acne Outbreaks
- Abdominal Pain
- Worsening Asthma Symptoms
- Worsening Signs and Symptoms of Irritable Bowel Syndrome
- Palpitations
- Acid Reflux

Nurses affected by bullying also may develop marital and intimate relationship problems as they bring the stress evoked by the bullying and incivility home. By isolating and not discussing what is going on at work, nurses' intimate partners (i.e. spouses and significant others) are seeing changes in mood and behavior, but are unaware of the reason why these changes are occurring. The opposite can occur when nurses have developed the pattern of constantly bombarding their partners with stories of their maltreatment at work. Partners may feel helpless and powerless to defend them (affected nurses) and as a result become frustrated themselves with the stories of bullying. The latter can lead to arguments and place stress on nurses' intimate relationships outside of work. It is important that nurses recognize signs and symptoms of their bullying impacting the intimate relationships they have with significant others. The following are signs and symptoms of strained intimate relationships secondary to bullying:

Signs and Symptoms of Strained Intimate Relationships Impacted by Bullying

- Mood Lability
- Disrupted Sleep and Rest Patterns
- Anger
- Isolation
- Frustration
- Bitterness
- Sexual Dysfunction
- Difficulty Concentrating
- Depression
- Difficulty Remembering and Recalling Day-to-Day Events
- Anxiety
- Fear

Nurses can learn to progress beyond the pain of bullying in their intimate relationships, by protectively, limiting the amount of information provided to their partners about the actual bullying taking place in the workplace. If this approach is taken, nurses must ensure that they have a close friend, therapist or counselor to still confide within. Without the support of others, these signs and symptoms can overwhelm nurses and impact not only their productivity at work, but their overall ability to function in their daily lives.

Making the Positive From the Negative

Nurses that have been affected by bullying have a difficult time feeling positive about their workplace. For some nurses, even driving by, entering the grounds or building where they work, can bring about feelings of anxiety, disgust, and frustration. It is important for nurses experiencing bullying to understand that the actual workplace itself is not causing harm to them, but the person(s) perpetuating the bullying are.

In order to maintain health and well-being, nurses affected by bullying must learn to recognize the value of positivity in their life. The workplace may be negative at this time because of the perpetrator, but the affected nurse's life is not all negative. By being able to differentiate between the emotional effects of dealing with incivility in the work environment versus the emotional issues in one's home life and other areas of their private life (i.e. friendships, church, etc.), the nurse is more likely to maintain a work-life balance.

For nurses struggling with the ability to acknowledge the positive in their lives, they may benefit from practicing positive affirmations and mindfulness. Practicing mindfulness can help nurses affected by bullying, to be thankful for their daily lives and the people and objects (i.e. flowers) that bring meaning to their lives. Positive affirmations can help nurses learn to change the words they use daily from negative to positive. Acknowledging the positive can help nurses mentally, emotionally, and spiritually, defeat the negative impact of bullies.

Protecting Future Generations of Nurses

The protection of future generations of nurses from incivility within the workplace begins with the acknowledgement that there is a problem of bullying in the nursing profession. The historical adage of *nurses eating their young* is not a normal expectation for men and woman entering the profession to experience. Nurses, theoretically, have no reason to uphold the standard of harming newer members of the profession.

The adage of *nurses eating their young*, has been equated with new nurses being initiated by older nurses to the profession. This initiation may involve the assignment of a complex patient assignment with the expectation to step up and handle the complex assignment independently, or fall apart under the pressure. Those nurses unable to thrive and survive this initiation, are seen as weak by their nursing colleagues perpetuating this behavior, and may be bullied as a result.

Allowing this unhealthy initiation of young nurses into the profession, is wrong. When nurses experience being treated unfairly by their colleagues, they too are more likely to repeat these behaviors with other nurses. Therefore, it is imperative that all nurses be accountable for maintaining civility within the workplace. This can be accomplished by following the American Association of Nursing Code of Ethics for the profession and the code's mandates for professional behavior within the workplace.

How Can I Help New Nurses Thrive?

Experienced nurses can assist new nurses and student nurses to thrive in the clinical environment by teaching them the value of respect, compassion, and kindness. The words respect, compassion, and kindness are not new to the nursing profession. These are words introduced in nursing school in foundational theoretical core courses, to help nursing students understanding the importance of valuing human life in the care of patients. These words are used in the evaluation and assessment of nursing students in the clinical environment to ensure that student nurses are able not only to just apply classroom theory, but application to practice. Caritas after all, is the foundation of the nursing profession. We provide help to others, ill strangers, because we care.

Because the concept of bullying is unfortunately, not new to the nursing profession, it is important that nursing students learn about this problem while within the academic setting. For nursing as a profession to become committed to developing a zero tolerance for bullying, nursing students must be taught that uncivil behaviors toward others in the classroom and workplace in unacceptable. Hence, nurse educators and clinical faculty must model civility for student nurses.

Civility can be introduced into the classroom environment through the development of curriculums that integrate the importance of nurses exhibiting professionalism, collegiality, courteousness, and respect. When civility is taught as a behavioral expectation for nursing classroom and the clinical environments, and these behavioral expectations are acknowledged in students' evaluations/assessments, the seriousness of the problem of incivility will be addressed. Below are examples of civility that can be taught by nurse educators within the classroom and clinical environments.

Activity One: Classroom Civility

Directions: As your professor discusses each topic, in groups of five, answer the questions and consider how incivility impacts you and your peers within your group. After 15 minutes of group discussion, report your findings to the class.

1. What is incivility?
    a. Define the word incivility
    b. Differentiate between the words civility and incivility
2. How does incivility present itself in the classroom?
    a. Students
    b. Professors

3. Have you ever witnessed a fellow nursing student bully a peer or a professor?
    a. Describe your reaction
    b. Discuss how you intervened or decided not to intervene

Activity Two- Civility in the Clinical Environment

Directions: As your professor discusses each topic, in groups of five, answer the questions and consider how incivility impacts you and your peers within your group. After 15 minutes of group discussion, report your findings to the class.

1. Have you ever experienced uncivil behaviors from a nurse or other health care professional?
    a. Describe the situation that the uncivil conduct was observed
    b. Consider if stress was a factor in the person not conducting themselves in a professional manner
2. If a nurse or other health care professional in the clinical environment has bullied you, have you reported their behavior to anyone?
    a. Informed your Clinical Professor
    b. Notified the unit manager
    c. Shared your concern with another nursing student
    d. Decided not to report the bullying
3. Do you feel that it is important to uphold the American Nurses Association's (ANA) Code of Ethics as it defines zero tolerance for workplace bullying?
    a. Explain how failure to uphold the ANA's stance on workplace bullying can impact nurses' care of patients
4. Can bullying impact the emotional, physical, and spiritual health of affected nurses?
    a. Describe a situation whereby you observed a nurse whose health was impacted by workplace bullying

By facilitating discussions within the classroom and clinical settings on incivility, prelicensure nursing students may be better prepared to address this workplace issue as it arises. Nursing students may also be more apt to, as licensed registered nurses, report perpetrators of workplace bullying. More importantly, patient safety and nurses' emotional and physical health will be maintained.

Nurse educators in the clinical and classroom settings, must themselves, be role models of civility. Failure to acknowledge and abstain from participation in uncivil behaviors demonstrates acceptance of incivility to students. The latter is unacceptable and means that faculty themselves are in violation of the ANA Code of Ethics.

Re-Owning You

Most nurses affected by bullying cannot say exactly when it occurred, but somewhere along the way, they lost themselves. By losing oneself, there may have been a change in nurses' levels of confidence, self-esteem, perceptions of their own academic and professional abilities, and even how affected nurses perceive their own physical beauty. The destruction done to nurses' spirits, emotions, and body require time to heal.

Nurses must understand the importance of recognizing the changes in themselves after being bullied in the workplace. Along with the changes in self-esteem and self-concept, relationships with family members and close friends may have been strained because of affected nurses becoming isolative or exhibiting labile moods, secondary to the effects of bullying. It may be necessary for affected nurses to receive counseling or therapy to discuss in private, what they have experienced.

Re-owning yourself, the person before the bullying and after the bullying, is necessary to evolve into a stronger person. Learning to embrace your faults and strengths, as well as your ability to overcome negativity displayed by others and directed toward you, provides the perspective of an overcomer. Nurses that have withstood the negativity of bullying have overcome falsehoods perpetrated against them and know how to survive personal attacks on their character.

Nurses that recover from bullying are those that are able to balance the forgiveness of their perpetrators, while no longer tolerating negative attacks against themselves. These nurses are also empowered to help others experiencing bullying in the workplace. Armed with the knowledge and experience of the detrimental effects of workplace bullying, victims are no longer victimized and can help change workplace cultures and policies to ensure that a zero tolerance of bullying and incivility exists.

Changing Your Outlook

The world can seem very different to nurses that have experienced bullying in the workplace. Nurses affected by bullying may become less trusting of others and cautious in developing relationships. Their outlook on life may change. This change comes about as a result of having experienced deception by perpetrators.

It is important that nurses change their outlook on life after the bullying experience for the better. While being bullied is painful, it does not define you nor does it prevent you from achieving greater success than you had before being bullied, after the bullying has ended. When victims change their outlook on the bullying experience, they change their pathway to veer toward success.

So, what does it mean to change one's outlook? Changing one's outlook can occur when someone decides after a negative experience such as a layoff from a job, that they will not allow the situation they have been placed within, to define them. The layoff then becomes an unexpected opportunity to retrain, go back to school or find a better position that can lead to further professional growth. The situation of the layoff has not immediately changed, but the way the person views the layoff has. Changing your outlook therefore is an opportunity to seek the positive in difficult situations, believing that change will come, despite the current situation.

In Search of Obstacles

An obstacle is a deterrent or something placed in one's way to impede progression. For nurses that have experienced bullying, they themselves can become their own obstacle. The hypervigilance that occurs while being bullied, brings about a sense of heightened awareness to one's emotions being potentially damaged by the perpetrator(s) or others. Nurses that have experienced physical threats of harm from perpetrators may develop tension in their posture resulting in muscular pain in their neck and back. Some nurses affected by bullying may had experienced being set-up by a perpetrator in a clinical environment, or being mobbed in a meeting by multiple perpetrators verbalizing negativities in attempt to discredit the affected nurse. The latter experience can cause affected nurses to struggle with self-confidence and experience paranoia because they feel unsafe in their workplace environment.

The multiple exposures to the unprovoked physical and emotional pain of bullying, can rob affected nurses of their peace and joy. Nurses must therefore be in-tuned to or made aware of mentally placing obstacles such as fear in front of their lives that cause them to miss opportunities to change careers, take risks, and meet new people. Remember, being bullied does not define who you are, nor what you will become. For nurses that have been bullied, growing from the experience provides them an opportunity to create their own path and help in the healing process of others because they themselves, have overcome a difficult situation.

Workplace Incivility in Healthcare

Workplace incivility can occur among any persons in healthcare. Be it manager-to nurse, patient-to-nurse, healthcare provider-to-nurse, nurse-to-nurse, or the involvement of other health care disciplines, incivility creates unhealthy workplaces. Unfortunately, the most common type of workplace incivility involving nurses, is nurse-to-nurse incivility (Frederick, 2014; Hoffman & Chunta, 2015).

In previous chapters, we discussed how turnover intentions and sick calls can be associated with bullying in the workplace. During times of nursing shortages in both clinical and academic settings, resolution to the issue of workplace incivility is vital to the health and well-being of nurses, and the patients in their care. It imperative that nurses become advocates for the American Nurses Association's stance on zero tolerance for incivility.

By becoming advocates in the promotion of workplace civility, nurses can help introduce work-based policies that will uphold zero tolerance. Nurse educators can help develop simulations that address incivility within the workplace. Clinical nurses can hold forums to promote open conversations among nurses and other professions, about the physiological and psychological dangers of workplace incivility and bullying. Self-help groups can be developed so that nurses affected by bullying have a safe and confidential place to share their stories and begin the healing process.

Moving Toward Resolution

In closing, examples of starting a self-help group, simulations, and developing forums in the workplace will be provided. The purpose of the presentation of these ideas at the end of this book is to help empower nurses to help one another and the profession. When we educate one another to the existence of workplace bullying within our profession, we can keep patients safe, improve the physical and mental health of nurses, and potentially, prevent a nurse from committing suicide.

SELF-HELP GROUPS

Purpose of Self-Help Groups

The purpose of self-help groups are to bring persons with the same or similar experiences together to provide support to one another. The difference between a self-help group versus group therapy, is that the group leader may not have a license in a mental health field, nor have formal training in the leading of a group. Self-help groups are peer-led and decisions are made with input from all group members.

Self-help groups can be beneficial for nurses experiencing bullying because these groups bring a group of nurses together that have all experienced some degree of workplace incivility. Nurses starting a self-help group of this kind, should chose a location whereby all members feel safe and that what they disclose will be kept confidential. Therefore, holding the group off of hospital other health care facilities, university, or college grounds is recommended. Do not use a group member's home, this can interfere with work-life balance. Instead, inquire about availability of space within a local library, community center, or church with ease of travel distance for group members.

Nurses participating in a self-help group do not have to write their names, nor contact information in a log or sign a contractual agreement. Confidentiality and anonymity should be maintained. Remember, the purpose of the group is for nurses being bullied at work, to receive support. Decide if the group will be left open for ongoing growth of membership, or closed when a designated number of nurse attendees is met. Also, consider if a determined amount of weeks (i.e. 6 weeks) for group sessions is indicated versus weekly or every-other-week attendance.

Nurses choosing to run a self-help group providing support to victims of bullying, should consider consulting someone that has expertise in the subject matter. Also, becoming a well-read learner about the topic of bullying and sharing the literature and resources with other members, can help participants empower themselves to change their situation. Group participants should help in the development of group rules, this will help members collaborate together and encourage group cohesiveness. Examples of group rules are below.

Group Rules

1. Information that is shared in the group must remain confidential
2. Avoid interrupting one another
3. Be respectful in all communications with one another
4. No yelling, cursing, or forceful physical touch is allowed
5. Empower and validate one another
6. If someone arrives late to the group, be courteous and do not disrupt the flow of the group conversations
7. Everyone has a voice and deserves to be heard and listened to
8. Seek opportunities to give thanks
9. Be respectful of other's beliefs even if they are different from your own
10. Be authentically you, while embracing the stronger person you are becoming

Pledges or Prayers

The development of a group pledge or prayer can be beneficial in bringing cohesiveness among group members. For example, the Serenity Prayer, written by theologian Reinhold Niebuhr (Sifton, 2005) in 1943 for his sermon in a New England church, is often associated with the self-help group, Alcoholics Anonymous. Whether you choose to adapt a pre-existing pledge or prayer, or develop your own, ensure that members are in agreement in the decision.

EXAMPLE OF WORKPLACE BULLYING SELF-HELP PLEDGE AND PRAYER

Anti-Bullying Nurses' Pledge

I resolve to look beyond the names that I have been called and see myself as a competent, intelligent, and worthy nurse. The bitter words of the bully, have no power over me. I stand strong and undefeated.

I will take care of my mental and physical well-being. I will take care of, enjoy quality time with, and love my family (and close friends). I will not allow the words of another to destroy my health, nor define who I am.

I will not allow my anger or hatred of the bully to interfere with my own blessings. I will demonstrate kindness and care to others and enjoy my life.

Anti-Bullying Nurses' Prayer

God, I know that you hear my prayer. I know that you feel my anguish over negative words spoken to me by a bully. I kneel in prayer to ask for your help, knowing that you will give it to me.

Free me from my frustration. Help me to concentrate and get my work done, to keep my patients safe from harm related to a distracted mind. Keep my mind dwelling upon all that is peaceful and calm in you.

Give me a voice and courageousness to speak boldly of what is right and just in order that I might end bullying not just for myself, but other nurses.

Nurse Development of Anti-Bully Forums

Forums are meetings within a designated place and time, meant to facilitate an exchange of ideas. Forums can be held online or in-person. Nurses can educate their colleagues and administration on the issue of workplace incivility through the use of forums. Whether a forum is developed online or for an in-person meeting, the topic with learning objectives must be developed. The facilitator(s) should be organized and have an understanding of the topic being presented.

Anti-bullying forums should balance times between questions being posed for discussion and participants (and facilitator(s)) providing feedback. Rules for respectful communication must be set before the forum begins. Also, the nurse facilitating the forum would benefit from having a co-facilitator to keep track of timing of the discussions and assist in the documenting of ideas. Ensure that participants that proposed ideas are given credit not only during the actual forum, but after. Participant ideas should be compiled and listed with their names credited. The latter builds cohesiveness and team building that can ultimately help drive policy development for workplace incivility at health care facilities at which the nurses work.

The following are examples of forum topics for discussions on workplace incivility:

(1). Bullying in the Workplace Harms More Than Just the One Person, (2). I Never Thought A Nurse Would Self-Harm Because of Bullying, (3). No One Deserves Emotional and Physical Pain in the Workplace, and (4). My Distraction Related to Being Bullied, Could Harm My Patients. Once a topic is selected, nurses organizing the forum should conduct a literature review. Once the literature review is completed, a proposal can be written in preparation for presentation to key stakeholders at participant nurses' workplaces (i.e. manager, director, and administration), based on the hierarchy set by their facility.

Forums can be a non-threatening way to begin the difficult conversation on the complex topic of workplace bullying. Nurses organizing the forum(s) can use compiled data to formulate policy for the development of healthy workplaces with zero tolerance for workplace bullying. Forums are another means to educate others on why workplace bullying is unhealthy.

USING SIMULATION TO TEACH NURSES ABOUT WORKPLACE INCIVILITY

Simulation

Simulation scenarios are used to present realistic situations in a safe environment, to facilitate learning. Simulations can be developed in academic, hospital, and other health care environments, to teach nurses how to handle incivility in the workplace. Nurse educators and Simulation Coordinators skilled in the development of simulation scenarios, can use this innovation to teach nurses how to recognize bullying, passive-aggressive behaviors, and verbal and nonverbal presentations of incivility.

The simulation scenarios can incorporate different situations that nurses could experience during workplace bullying. Small groups of nurses (no more than 3 or 4 per scenario) participate in the actual simulation itself and sign consent forms to give permission for the simulation to be taped so that it can be viewed by their participant group during debriefing. During debriefing, the groups of nurses discuss what occurred during the workplace incivility scenario and how each situation could have been dealt with.

Four simulations will be provided as examples of scenarios that nurses in a variety of work settings, can adapt to their staff's specific issues and needs.

Remember, the purpose of the simulation scenario is to promote education and discussion on how to cope with and end workplace bullying. Nurses developing simulations should use current evidenced-based practice articles addressing each scenario as the foundation of the simulation development. Thorough research of each simulation scenario brings about understanding of the topic for participants, and promotes a deeper level of thinking about the topic (i.e. socratic learning).

SIMULATION SCENARIOS

Simulation 1: "Oh, Did You Say Something?"

- **Scenario Setting:** Academia, a meeting involving nursing professors.
- **Roles Assigned:** Dr. Miles, 5 to 6 professors, 1 Department Chair

Learning Objectives

1. Identify the professors exhibiting incivility.
2. Describe the forms of workplace incivility being expressed by the professors.
3. Determine the normalcy of Dr. Miles' response to her colleagues' behaviors.
4. Discuss why the six professors did not support Dr. Miles.
5. Consider why the Department Chair failed to intervene and potentially end the bullying behaviors.

Background Information

Nursing Professor Audrey Miles has just been awarded a grant for 1 million dollars for research on Lyme disease. The grant is interdisciplinary and involves the collaboration of a biology professor and a psychology professor.

Scenario Begins

The nursing professors enter an empty conference room and begin to sit down. The Department Chair makes the announcement that Dr. Miles and her colleagues have just been awarded a research grant for 1 million dollars. In a room of 25 professors, 6 professors clap and offer congratulations while

19 professors remain silent. The Department Chair chooses to ignore what has occurred.

As the meeting progresses, whenever Dr. Miles speaks, side conversations are started and the 19 professors pretend as if she is not talking at all. The meeting progresses and one of the 6 supportive faculty says to Dr. Miles, "How will you incorporate your research findings into your work with the nursing students?"

Dr. Miles explains that she will be teaching in addition to her Community Health course, a new course that she is developing that addresses global health and disease. A professor then says to Dr. Miles, "Do you really think a global health class is needed? When did you as a community health nurse become an expert on global health? What do you know?"

As Dr. Miles attempts to answer her colleagues' questions, she is bombarded by verbal attacks on her expertise as an academic and her knowledge of global health by different professors. She is shocked by their blatant disrespect of her and their unprofessional behavior. She sits in silence as the mean comments continue and the other 6 professors and Department Chair look on.

Debrief

Discussions will focus on the definition of a mob in incivility. A mob constitutes a group of persons who seek to discredit and bully their target. In this case, Dr. Miles was the target. The likely cause of the bullying was professional jealousy.

SIMULATION SCENARIOS

Simulation 2: "You Really Don't Know How to Do This?"

- **Scenario Setting:** Clinical Unit, Surgery Service Line.
- **Roles Assigned:** 2 Registered Nurses and 1 Patient

Learning Objectives

1. Determine if poor communication was a factor in how the nurse treated Ben.
2. Discuss how Ben's silence in not addressing the patient's concern, impacted the nurse-patient relationship.

Background Information

A graduate nurse has only used a Smart Pump new to the facility, once. He is preparing to hang an antibiotic to be administered intravenously (IV) on a primary continuous line and asks a colleague for assistance.

Scenario Begins

New graduate nurse Ben approaches one of his senior colleagues and requests assistance with using a new Smart Pump to administer the IV antibiotic piperacillin tazobactam (Zosyn). The nurse agrees to assist Ben and accompanies him to his patient's hospital room.

Ben introduces his colleague to the patient and explains the procedure and that his colleague will be assisting him. As Ben's colleague explained each step in the use of the new Smart Pump to him, she would make a sarcastic comment about his inexperience as a new graduate nurse. As the medication began to infuse into the patient's peripheral IV, the nurse stated, "Ben, so glad I was able to help. I would not want to risk you harming a patient."

The patient looked terrified. As the more senior nurse exits the room, the patient asks the nurse, "Can you be my nurse tonight?" The nurse agrees and Ben appears embarrassed and hurt.

When the nurses walk out of the patient's room, Ben asks the nurse, "Why did you say that." The nurse responds, "It's true. You have no idea what you are doing."

Debrief

Discuss how the senior nurse's comments impacted Ben's nurse-patient relationship. What could Ben have said to the patient to address the patient's concerns about his level of experience as a nurse? What would you do?

SIMULATION SCENARIOS

Simulation 3: "Am I Supposed to Read Your Mind!"

- **Scenario Setting:** Clinical Unit, Medicine Service Line.
- **Roles Assigned:** 1 Registered Nurse and 1 Healthcare Provider

Learning Objectives

1. Discuss if the nurse should be held accountable for awakening the sleeping healthcare provider.
2. Consider the appropriateness of the healthcare provider's response.
3. Determine if this interaction constitutes bullying.

Background Information

Mary is a healthcare provider that is on her third night as the on-call provider for the Medicine Service Line. There have been several sick calls by her peers related to a norovirus that was on one of the units, so she has to cover.

Scenario Begins

It has been a very busy evening on the Medical Unit. Rachel, one of the nurses, has just admitted her third patient in four hours, while maintaining a patient assignment of four patients, one of whom is receiving a blood transfusion. Rachel has just completed the nursing assessment of one of her admissions when she hears someone yell out, "Help me!"

Rachel finds one of her newly admitted patients on the floor. The patient has no visible injuries, but reports that he may have hit his head slightly on the corner of the hospital bed. Rachel, while assessing the patient, notices a small laceration at the top of his head. The patient denies pain and keeps assuring Rachel that he is fine.

Rachel has a colleague sit with the patient on the floor in his room where he was found, and calls the healthcare provider. The healthcare provider answers the phone and says, "This better be important, I just finished all of the new admissions orders and fell asleep." Rachel explains that one of the new admissions had a fall in their hospital room, but is denying pain and his vital signs are stable.

The healthcare provider interrupts Rachel as she explains that she noted a small laceration on the top of his head and says, "Sounds like this can wait until the morning." The healthcare provider then hangs up the phone. Rachel calls the provider back and says, "Why did you hang up on me. I am just calling to request a computed tomography scan (CT scan) to ensure that my patient does not have a head injury."

The provider, angered by the nurse's response says, "I will come and see your patient Rachel and order a CT scan. I also plan to report you for insubordination to your nurse manager. You should not have hung up on me."

Debrief

Determine were there any issues with the communications that occurred between the two health care professionals. Discuss if it was appropriate for the nurse to have awakened the healthcare provider. Consider what approaches could have been taken and done differently by the nurse and provider.

SIMULATION SCENARIOS

Simulation 4: "I Am Not Your Servant."

- **Scenario Setting:** Outpatient Clinic, Patient incivility directed at an ethnic-minority nurse.
- **Roles Assigned:** 1 Patient and 1 Nurse

Learning Objectives

1. Explain if the nurse experienced discrimination.
2. Consider the necessity of working in workplaces that demonstrate cultural awareness and sensitivity.
3. Discuss if this interaction between the nurse and patient constitutes bullying.

Background Information

A nurse working in a community clinic is completing an intake on a patient scheduled for his yearly physical examination. The nurse is a native of Lagos, a city in Nigeria who is an American citizen and has lived in the United States for 10 years.

Scenario Begins

The nurse enters the clinic waiting room and calls the patient's full name. The patient slowly approaches the nurse and says, "Is it me you that you called young lady?" The nurse verifies the patient's name and confirms the patient's medical record number. The nurse acknowledges the patient by nodding her head and states, "Nice to meet you."

The nurse escorts the patient to an examination room and begins to ask the patient to change into a disposable gown. She provides privacy for the patient to change and returns to the examination room. The nurse explains to the patient, "I will be performing a physical assessment and then obtain your weight. Let's begin with some general questions about how you have been feeling overall."

The patient looked puzzled at the nurse. Then stated, "Hold on. I am liberated and all, but you aren't a nurse and definitely not a doctor. You will not be examining me. You're just an aide." The nurse had an identification badge that had her picture, name, and title displayed on it. She showed the patient the badge and reassured the patient that she was capable of performing the care of which she had discussed.

The patient became angry and stated, "In the United States we do not allow anyone to just come off some boat and give us care. How do I know that you do not have Ebola." The nurse said calmly to the patient, "I have shown you nothing but respect. I am actually a doctor in my own country. I will talk to my nurse manager to ensure that you receive the services of another nurse. Thank you." The nurse left the room and closed the door.

Debrief

Did the nurse handle the situation in a professional manner? If you were the nurse manager, how would you proceed with assigning the patient another nurse? Should the incident be discussed with the nurse? How about the patient? If yes, why? Is cultural awareness and sensitivity important in health care environments? Do you think this nurse was bullied or just disrespected?

REFERENCES

Berndsen, M., Wenzel, M., Thomas, E. F., & Noske, B. (2017). I feel you feel what I feel: Perceived perspective-taking promotes victims' conciliatory attitudes because of Inferred emotions in the offender. *European Journal of Social Psychology*, *48*(2), 103–120. doi:10.1002/ejsp.2321

Dzurec, L. C., Kennison, M., & Albataineh, R. (2014). Unacknowledged threats proffered "in a manner of speaking:" Recognizing workplace bullying as shaming. *Journal of Nursing Scholarship*, *46*(4), 281–291. doi:10.1111/jnu.12080 PMID:24754642

Enright, R. D., & Fitzgibbons, R. (2015). *Forgiveness therapy*. Washington, DC: APA Books.

Frederick, D. (n.d.). Bullying, mentoring, and patient care. *Association of Perioperative Registered Nurses Journal, 99*(5), 587-593.

Griffin, M., & Clark, C. (2014). Revisiting cognitive rehearsal as an intervention against incivility and lateral violence in nursing: 10 years later. *Journal of Continuing Education in Nursing, 45*(12), 535–542. doi:10.3928/00220124-20141122-02 PMID:25406637

Harris, A. H. S., & Thoresen, C. E. (2005). Forgiveness, unforgiveness, health and disease. In E. L. Worthington (Ed.), *Handbook of forgiveness* (pp. 321–334). New York, NY: Routledge Publishing.

Hoffman, R. L., & Chunta, K. (2015). Workplace incivility: Promoting zero tolerance in nursing. *Journal of Radiology Nursing, 34*(4), 222–227. doi:10.1016/j.jradnu.2015.09.004

Littlejohn, P. (2012). The missing link: Using emotional intelligence to reduce workplace and workplace violence in our nursing and other health care professions. *Journal of Professional Nursing, 28*(6), 360–368. doi:10.1016/j.profnurs.2012.04.006 PMID:23158199

Mayo Clinic. (2015). *Mindfulness exercises: See how mindfulness helps you to live in the moment.* Retrieved from http://www.mayoclinic.org/healthy-lifestyle/consumer-health/in-depth/mindfulness-exercises/art-20046356

McCance, K. L., & Huether, S. E. (2018). *Pathophysiology: The biologic basis for disease in Adults and children* (8th ed.). New York, NY: Elsevier Health Sciences.

Meires, J. (2018). Workplace incivility. The Essentials: Using emotional intelligence to curtail bullying in the workplace. *Urologic Nursing, 38*(3), 150–153. doi:10.7257/1053-816X.2018.38.3.150

Rodwell, J., & Demir, D. (2012). Psychological consequences of bullying for hospital and aged-care nurses. *International Nursing Review, 59*(4), 539–546. doi:10.1111/j.1466-7657.2012.01018.x PMID:23134139

Salovey, P., & Mayer, J. D. (1990). Emotional intelligence. *Imagination, Cognition and Personality, 9*(3), 185–211. doi:10.2190/DUGG-P24E-52WK-6CDG

Seedall, R. B., Butler, M. H., & Elledge, J. Z. (2014). Does religious motivation influence the conceptualization and acceptability of forgiveness as a therapeutic intervention? *The American Journal of Family Therapy*, *42*(2), 127–140. doi:10.1080/01926187.2013.772868

Sifton, E. (2005). *The serenity prayer: Faith and politics in times of peace and war*. New York, NY: W. W Norton Company.

Strelan, P., Di Fiore, C., & Prooijen, J.-W. V. (2017). The empowering effect of punishment on forgiveness. *European Journal of Social Psychology*, *47*(4), 472–487. doi:10.1002/ejsp.2254

The Joint Commission. (2016). *Quick Safety 24: Bullying has no place in health care*. Retrieved from https://www.jointcommission.org/issues/article.aspx?Article=rFhOFvmOhideyaeaXWHwdF7iIsdGP+TcEobEhA7d2RU=

Toussaint, L. L., Williams, D. R., Musick, M. A., & Everson, S. A. (2001). Forgiveness and Health: Age differences in a U.S. probability sample. *Journal of Adult Development*, *8*(4), 249–257. doi:10.1023/A:1011394629736

Vliet Van, K. J. (2008). Shame and resilience in adulthood: A grounded theory study. *Journal of Counseling Psychology*, *55*(2), 233–245. doi:10.1037/0022-0167.55.2.233

Williams, M., & Penman, D. (2012). *Mindfulness: An Eight-Week Plan for Finding Peace in A Frantic World*. New York, NY: Rodale, Inc.

Appendix

ORIGINAL ARTWORK AND PHOTOGRAPHS

All paintings and drawings are original art work created by artist, E. Green. The male and female silhouettes were drawn by Joshua William Green. Photographs were taken by Cheryl Ann Green.

Related Readings

To continue IGI Global's long-standing tradition of advancing innovation through emerging research, please find below a compiled list of recommended IGI Global book chapters and journal articles in the areas of nursing, workplace bullying, and workplace culture. These related readings will provide additional information and guidance to further enrich your knowledge and assist you with your own research.

Akca, M., & Çalışkan, B. Ö. (2018). Gender Diversity in Board of Directors: A Content Analysis From Turkey – Women's Presence Level in Turkey's Boards. In N. Sharma, V. Singh, & S. Pathak (Eds.), *Management Techniques for a Diverse and Cross-Cultural Workforce* (pp. 20–38). Hershey, PA: IGI Global. doi:10.4018/978-1-5225-4933-8.ch002

Al-Huneiti, R., Hunaiti, Z., Al-Masaeed, S., Balachandran, W., & Mansour, E. (2016). Nurses' Attitudes Towards E-Learning for E-health Education. *International Journal of Handheld Computing Research*, *7*(1), 77–84. doi:10.4018/IJHCR.2016010104

Angelova, R. A. (2017). Cross-Cultural Management of the European Textile and Clothing Industries: Application of Hofstede's Cultural Dimensions. In B. Christiansen & H. Chandan (Eds.), *Handbook of Research on Organizational Culture and Diversity in the Modern Workforce* (pp. 239–260). Hershey, PA: IGI Global. doi:10.4018/978-1-5225-2250-8.ch011

Athota, V. S. (2017). Foundations and Future of Well-Being: How Personality Influences Happiness and Well-Being. In S. Háša & R. Brunet-Thornton (Eds.), *Impact of Organizational Trauma on Workplace Behavior and Performance* (pp. 279–294). Hershey, PA: IGI Global. doi:10.4018/978-1-5225-2021-4.ch012

Bingham, H. M. (2017). Undergraduate Nursing Curriculum Content Focuses on Emerging Issues that Influence Health. In M. Smith & A. Jury (Eds.), *Workforce Development Theory and Practice in the Mental Health Sector* (pp. 182–199). Hershey, PA: IGI Global. doi:10.4018/978-1-5225-1874-7.ch009

Bishop, J. (2017). Detecting Sexual Harassment in Workplace Electronic Communications Networks: The Role of "PROTEGER" for Augmentive Behaviour Monitoring. In B. Christiansen & H. Chandan (Eds.), *Handbook of Research on Organizational Culture and Diversity in the Modern Workforce* (pp. 181–216). Hershey, PA: IGI Global. doi:10.4018/978-1-5225-2250-8.ch009

Byrd-Poller, L., Farmer, J. L., & Ford, V. (2017). The Role of Leaders in Facilitating Healing After Organizational Trauma. In S. Háša & R. Brunet-Thornton (Eds.), *Impact of Organizational Trauma on Workplace Behavior and Performance* (pp. 318–340). Hershey, PA: IGI Global. doi:10.4018/978-1-5225-2021-4.ch014

Cejka, P., & Mohelska, H. (2017). National Culture Influence on Organisational Trauma: A Conceptual Framework Review. In S. Háša & R. Brunet-Thornton (Eds.), *Impact of Organizational Trauma on Workplace Behavior and Performance* (pp. 162–186). Hershey, PA: IGI Global. doi:10.4018/978-1-5225-2021-4.ch007

Chaudhary, N. S., & Yadav, R. (2018). Cross-Cultural Conflicts: Concept, Causes, and Elucidations. In N. Sharma, V. Singh, & S. Pathak (Eds.), *Management Techniques for a Diverse and Cross-Cultural Workforce* (pp. 79–96). Hershey, PA: IGI Global. doi:10.4018/978-1-5225-4933-8.ch005

Choi, Y. (2018). A Study on the Prevention of Cyberbullying in Workplaces. *International Journal of Technoethics*, *9*(1), 18–26. doi:10.4018/IJT.2018010102

Choi, Y. (2019). Workplace Violence and Social Engineering Among Korean Employees. *International Journal of Asian Business and Information Management*, *10*(1), 26–37. doi:10.4018/IJABIM.2019010102

Chou, P. (2018). Workplace Social Support and Attitude toward Enterprise Resource Planning System: A Perspective of Organizational Change. *International Journal of Information Systems and Social Change*, *9*(1), 58–76. doi:10.4018/IJISSC.2018010104

Cicerali, E. E., & Cicerali, L. K. (2017). Workplace Incivility as Low-Level Violence: Theories, Consequences, and Future Research Suggestions. In B. Christiansen & H. Chandan (Eds.), *Handbook of Research on Organizational Culture and Diversity in the Modern Workforce* (pp. 155–180). Hershey, PA: IGI Global. doi:10.4018/978-1-5225-2250-8.ch008

Cleve, R. A., Işık, İ., & Pecanha, V. D. (2017). Sexual Identities in the Workplace: Avoiding Organizational Trauma When Disclosure Occurs – Current Perspectives. In S. Háša & R. Brunet-Thornton (Eds.), *Impact of Organizational Trauma on Workplace Behavior and Performance* (pp. 188–220). Hershey, PA: IGI Global. doi:10.4018/978-1-5225-2021-4.ch008

Cordeiro, C. M. (2017). Relativity in Perspective in Culture Theories: The Götheborg IV Model. In B. Christiansen & H. Chandan (Eds.), *Handbook of Research on Organizational Culture and Diversity in the Modern Workforce* (pp. 217–238). Hershey, PA: IGI Global. doi:10.4018/978-1-5225-2250-8.ch010

Das, R. (2018). Human Resource Management in Indian Microfinance Institutions. In N. Sharma, V. Singh, & S. Pathak (Eds.), *Management Techniques for a Diverse and Cross-Cultural Workforce* (pp. 297–311). Hershey, PA: IGI Global. doi:10.4018/978-1-5225-4933-8.ch017

de Soir, E., & Kleber, R. (2017). Understanding the Core of Psychological Trauma: Trauma in Contemporary French Theory. In S. Háša & R. Brunet-Thornton (Eds.), *Impact of Organizational Trauma on Workplace Behavior and Performance* (pp. 57–75). Hershey, PA: IGI Global. doi:10.4018/978-1-5225-2021-4.ch003

Dunlap, R. K., & Morse, E. A. (2018). Refugee Families and Undergraduate Nursing Service-Learning: Thinking Globally, Acting Locally. In O. Delano-Oriaran, M. Penick-Parks, & S. Fondrie (Eds.), *Culturally Engaging Service-Learning With Diverse Communities* (pp. 248–265). Hershey, PA: IGI Global. doi:10.4018/978-1-5225-2900-2.ch015

Eckardt, P., Janotha, B., Marino, M. A., Erlanger, D. P., & Cannella, D. (2016). Equipping Advanced Practice Nurses with Real-World Skills. In Y. Rosen, S. Ferrara, & M. Mosharraf (Eds.), *Handbook of Research on Technology Tools for Real-World Skill Development* (pp. 163–189). Hershey, PA: IGI Global. doi:10.4018/978-1-4666-9441-5.ch007

Efeoğlu, E. I., & Pekkan, N. U. (2017). The Relationship Between Employee Empowerment and Organizational Cynicism: An Implementation in the Banking Sector. In B. Christiansen & H. Chandan (Eds.), *Handbook of Research on Organizational Culture and Diversity in the Modern Workforce* (pp. 309–322). Hershey, PA: IGI Global. doi:10.4018/978-1-5225-2250-8.ch014

Fahlman, D. W. (2017). Reflections on Distributive Leadership for Work-Based Mobile Learning of Canadian Registered Nurses. *International Journal of Mobile and Blended Learning*, *9*(3), 1–11. doi:10.4018/IJMBL.2017070101

Ferrari, F. (2017). Human Resource Management and Organizational Reliability: Coordination Mechanisms, Training Models, and Diagnostic Systems for Contingency Management. In B. Christiansen & H. Chandan (Eds.), *Handbook of Research on Organizational Culture and Diversity in the Modern Workforce* (pp. 43–59). Hershey, PA: IGI Global. doi:10.4018/978-1-5225-2250-8.ch003

Gallego, J. (2017). Organizational Trauma and Change Management. In S. Háša & R. Brunet-Thornton (Eds.), *Impact of Organizational Trauma on Workplace Behavior and Performance* (pp. 140–161). Hershey, PA: IGI Global. doi:10.4018/978-1-5225-2021-4.ch006

Grandón, K. L., & Reinoso, L. A. (2016). Social Responsibility of Healthcare Organizations and the Role of the Nurse. In J. Saiz-Álvarez (Ed.), *Handbook of Research on Social Entrepreneurship and Solidarity Economics* (pp. 453–474). Hershey, PA: IGI Global. doi:10.4018/978-1-5225-0097-1.ch022

Greenfield, M. (2017). Perspectives on the Historical Evolution of the People Side of Business. In B. Christiansen & H. Chandan (Eds.), *Handbook of Research on Organizational Culture and Diversity in the Modern Workforce* (pp. 1–22). Hershey, PA: IGI Global. doi:10.4018/978-1-5225-2250-8.ch001

Gupta, M. (2018). Developing Strategic Leadership in the Indian Context: Leadership. In N. Sharma, V. Singh, & S. Pathak (Eds.), *Management Techniques for a Diverse and Cross-Cultural Workforce* (pp. 224–235). Hershey, PA: IGI Global. doi:10.4018/978-1-5225-4933-8.ch013

Habil, H., Othman, R., & Kahar, R. (2016). Nursing as a Global Career: Meeting the Challenges of the Profession from a Language for Specific Purposes (LSP) Perspective. *International Journal of Knowledge-Based Organizations*, *6*(4), 62–74. doi:10.4018/IJKBO.2016100106

Hameed, Z., Khan, I. U., Chudhery, M. A., & Ding, D. (2017). Incivility and Counterproductive Work Behavior: A Moderated Mediation Model of Emotional Regulation and Psychological Distress. *International Journal of Applied Behavioral Economics*, *6*(3), 1–22. doi:10.4018/IJABE.2017070101

Ifinedo, P. (2017). Using an Extended Theory of Planned Behavior to Study Nurses' Adoption of Healthcare Information Systems in Nova Scotia. *International Journal of Technology Diffusion*, *8*(1), 1–17. doi:10.4018/IJTD.2017010101

Isik, I. (2017). Organizations and Exposure to Trauma at a Collective Level: The Taxonomy of Potentially Traumatic Events. In S. Háša & R. Brunet-Thornton (Eds.), *Impact of Organizational Trauma on Workplace Behavior and Performance* (pp. 18–56). Hershey, PA: IGI Global. doi:10.4018/978-1-5225-2021-4.ch002

Itam, U., & Bagali, M. M. (2018). Diversity and Inclusion Management: A Focus on Employee Engagement. In N. Sharma, V. Singh, & S. Pathak (Eds.), *Management Techniques for a Diverse and Cross-Cultural Workforce* (pp. 149–171). Hershey, PA: IGI Global. doi:10.4018/978-1-5225-4933-8.ch009

Javaid, M. U., Isha, A. S., Nubling, M., Mirza, M. Z., & Ghazali, Z. (2017). Human Factors in Context to Occupational Health and Wellbeing. In B. Christiansen & H. Chandan (Eds.), *Handbook of Research on Organizational Culture and Diversity in the Modern Workforce* (pp. 60–77). Hershey, PA: IGI Global. doi:10.4018/978-1-5225-2250-8.ch004

Jeong, H. (2018). Nursing Students' Perception of Medical Information Protection in Hospitals. *International Journal of E-Health and Medical Communications*, *9*(4), 11–19. doi:10.4018/IJEHMC.2018100102

Jerabek, I., & Muoio, D. (2017). The Stress Profile: The Influence of Personal Characteristics on Response to Occupational Trauma. In S. Háša & R. Brunet-Thornton (Eds.), *Impact of Organizational Trauma on Workplace Behavior and Performance* (pp. 77–119). Hershey, PA: IGI Global. doi:10.4018/978-1-5225-2021-4.ch004

Jones, M., & Berhie, G. (2019). Efficacy of Telemedicine in Psychiatry and Mental Health Nursing. *International Journal of Extreme Automation and Connectivity in Healthcare*, *1*(1), 29–39. doi:10.4018/IJEACH.2019010104

Joshi, M. (2018). Workforce Trends and Challenges: A Peek Into the Future. In N. Sharma, V. Singh, & S. Pathak (Eds.), *Management Techniques for a Diverse and Cross-Cultural Workforce* (pp. 39–53). Hershey, PA: IGI Global. doi:10.4018/978-1-5225-4933-8.ch003

Kamasak, R., Kar, A., Yavuz, M., & Baykut, S. (2017). Qualitative Methods in Organizational Research: An Example of Grounded Theory Data Analysis. In B. Christiansen & H. Chandan (Eds.), *Handbook of Research on Organizational Culture and Diversity in the Modern Workforce* (pp. 23–42). Hershey, PA: IGI Global. doi:10.4018/978-1-5225-2250-8.ch002

Kamboj, S., & Sarmah, B. (2018). Antecedents and Consequences of Employee Engagement for a Diverse Workforce. In N. Sharma, V. Singh, & S. Pathak (Eds.), *Management Techniques for a Diverse and Cross-Cultural Workforce* (pp. 132–148). Hershey, PA: IGI Global. doi:10.4018/978-1-5225-4933-8.ch008

Karapinar, P. B., & Camgoz, S. M. (2017). Well-Being at Work: A Comprehensive Review About Its Predictors and Outcomes. In B. Christiansen & H. Chandan (Eds.), *Handbook of Research on Organizational Culture and Diversity in the Modern Workforce* (pp. 78–99). Hershey, PA: IGI Global. doi:10.4018/978-1-5225-2250-8.ch005

Kasemsap, K. (2017). Exploring the Role of Organizational Justice in the Modern Workplace. In B. Christiansen & H. Chandan (Eds.), *Handbook of Research on Organizational Culture and Diversity in the Modern Workforce* (pp. 323–345). Hershey, PA: IGI Global. doi:10.4018/978-1-5225-2250-8.ch015

Kasemsap, K. (2017). Mastering Employee Turnover Intention in the Modern Workforce. In B. Christiansen & H. Chandan (Eds.), *Handbook of Research on Organizational Culture and Diversity in the Modern Workforce* (pp. 382–401). Hershey, PA: IGI Global. doi:10.4018/978-1-5225-2250-8.ch018

Kılıç, B. (2017). An Organizational Trauma Intervention: A Case From Turkey. In S. Háša & R. Brunet-Thornton (Eds.), *Impact of Organizational Trauma on Workplace Behavior and Performance* (pp. 264–277). Hershey, PA: IGI Global. doi:10.4018/978-1-5225-2021-4.ch011

Kirschner, A., Kirschner, S., Seebauer, C., & Bethke, B. (2017). The Potential of Mobile Health in Nursing: The Use of Mobile Communication Technology in Plasma-Supported Outpatient Wound Care in Germany. *International Journal of Reliable and Quality E-Healthcare*, *6*(4), 49–58. doi:10.4018/IJRQEH.2017100106

Kučera, D. (2017). The Potential of Spirituality for the Treatment of Organizational Trauma. In S. Háša & R. Brunet-Thornton (Eds.), *Impact of Organizational Trauma on Workplace Behavior and Performance* (pp. 295–317). Hershey, PA: IGI Global. doi:10.4018/978-1-5225-2021-4.ch013

Kumar, R., & Jha, V. (2017). Traits of Leaders and Active Listening: A Theory. In B. Christiansen & H. Chandan (Eds.), *Handbook of Research on Organizational Culture and Diversity in the Modern Workforce* (pp. 364–381). Hershey, PA: IGI Global. doi:10.4018/978-1-5225-2250-8.ch017

Long, C. S. (2017). The Relationship Between Work-Life Balance (WLB) and Firm Performance. In B. Christiansen & H. Chandan (Eds.), *Handbook of Research on Organizational Culture and Diversity in the Modern Workforce* (pp. 402–411). Hershey, PA: IGI Global. doi:10.4018/978-1-5225-2250-8.ch019

McKeown, A. E. (2016). Nurses, Healthcare, and Environmental Pollution and Solutions: Breaking the Cycle of Harm. In A. McKeown & G. Bugyi (Eds.), *Impact of Water Pollution on Human Health and Environmental Sustainability* (pp. 174–197). Hershey, PA: IGI Global. doi:10.4018/978-1-4666-9559-7.ch008

Mehra, S., & Sharma, K. (2018). Diversity Management: A New Perspective. In N. Sharma, V. Singh, & S. Pathak (Eds.), *Management Techniques for a Diverse and Cross-Cultural Workforce* (pp. 1–19). Hershey, PA: IGI Global. doi:10.4018/978-1-5225-4933-8.ch001

Nandamuri, P. P., Mishra, M. K., & Ch, G. (2018). Relativity Applies to Physics, Not Ethics. In N. Sharma, V. Singh, & S. Pathak (Eds.), *Management Techniques for a Diverse and Cross-Cultural Workforce* (pp. 236–258). Hershey, PA: IGI Global. doi:10.4018/978-1-5225-4933-8.ch014

Nguyen, L., Wickramasinghe, N., Botti, M., Redley, B., Haddad, P., & Muhammad, I. (2017). Investigating Acceptance of Nursing Information Systems through UTAUT Lens. In N. Wickramasinghe (Ed.), *Handbook of Research on Healthcare Administration and Management* (pp. 349–368). Hershey, PA: IGI Global. doi:10.4018/978-1-5225-0920-2.ch020

Oliveira, D., Duarte, J., Abelha, A., & Machado, J. (2018). Step Towards Interoperability in Nursing Practice. *International Journal of Public Health Management and Ethics*, *3*(1), 26–37. doi:10.4018/IJPHME.2018010103

Orta, I. M., & Camgoz, S. M. (2017). Exploring Emotional Intelligence at Work: A Review of Current Evidence. In B. Christiansen & H. Chandan (Eds.), *Handbook of Research on Organizational Culture and Diversity in the Modern Workforce* (pp. 346–363). Hershey, PA: IGI Global. doi:10.4018/978-1-5225-2250-8.ch016

Oyarzun, B., & Gazza, E. A. (2017). Online Applied Learning in Nursing Education. In J. Stefaniak (Ed.), *Advancing Medical Education Through Strategic Instructional Design* (pp. 150–163). Hershey, PA: IGI Global. doi:10.4018/978-1-5225-2098-6.ch007

Pandey, S., & Sharma, V. (2016). Understanding Work-Related Stress, Job Conditions, Work Culture and Workaholism Phenomenon as Predictors of HR Crisis: An Empirical Study of the Indian IT Sector. *International Journal of Human Capital and Information Technology Professionals*, *7*(2), 68–80. doi:10.4018/IJHCITP.2016040105

Parmar, A. D., & Patel, C. (2018). Role of Team Climate in Improving Team Functioning and Team Empowerment. In N. Sharma, V. Singh, & S. Pathak (Eds.), *Management Techniques for a Diverse and Cross-Cultural Workforce* (pp. 186–205). Hershey, PA: IGI Global. doi:10.4018/978-1-5225-4933-8.ch011

Pavlovic, N. (2018). The Elements of Work Environment: Organizational Culture, Organizational Climate, and Job Satisfaction. In N. Sharma, V. Singh, & S. Pathak (Eds.), *Management Techniques for a Diverse and Cross-Cultural Workforce* (pp. 55–78). Hershey, PA: IGI Global. doi:10.4018/978-1-5225-4933-8.ch004

Pena, P. A., Van den Broucke, S., Sylin, M., Leysen, J., & de Soir, E. (2017). Definitions, Typologies, and Processes Involved in Organizational Trauma: A Literature Review. In S. Háša & R. Brunet-Thornton (Eds.), *Impact of Organizational Trauma on Workplace Behavior and Performance* (pp. 1–17). Hershey, PA: IGI Global. doi:10.4018/978-1-5225-2021-4.ch001

Priya, B., & Singh, V. (2018). Relationship Between Empowerment and Organizational Commitment: An Empirical Study of IT Industry. In N. Sharma, V. Singh, & S. Pathak (Eds.), *Management Techniques for a Diverse and Cross-Cultural Workforce* (pp. 172–185). Hershey, PA: IGI Global. doi:10.4018/978-1-5225-4933-8.ch010

Rajalakshmi, M., & Naresh, B. (2018). Influence of Cyber and Workplace Bullying Towards Employee Negative Emotions the Moderating Role of Gender. *International Journal of Cyber Behavior, Psychology and Learning*, *8*(2), 20–34. doi:10.4018/IJCBPL.2018040102

Rana, S. (2018). Performance Appraisal Techniques Across Various Sectors in India. In N. Sharma, V. Singh, & S. Pathak (Eds.), *Management Techniques for a Diverse and Cross-Cultural Workforce* (pp. 259–279). Hershey, PA: IGI Global. doi:10.4018/978-1-5225-4933-8.ch015

Rana, S., & Sharma, R. (2018). An Overview of Employer Branding With Special Reference to Indian Organizations. In N. Sharma, V. Singh, & S. Pathak (Eds.), *Management Techniques for a Diverse and Cross-Cultural Workforce* (pp. 116–131). Hershey, PA: IGI Global. doi:10.4018/978-1-5225-4933-8.ch007

Rexhepi, H., & Persson, A. (2017). Challenges to Implementing IT Support for Evidence Based Practice Among Nurses and Assistant Nurses: A Qualitative Study. *Journal of Electronic Commerce in Organizations*, *15*(2), 61–76. doi:10.4018/JECO.2017040105

Salazar, L. R. (2017). Workplace Bullying in Digital Environments: Antecedents, Consequences, Prevention, and Future Directions. In B. Christiansen & H. Chandan (Eds.), *Handbook of Research on Organizational Culture and Diversity in the Modern Workforce* (pp. 132–154). Hershey, PA: IGI Global. doi:10.4018/978-1-5225-2250-8.ch007

Salifu, S. (2017). A Blueprint for Online Licensed Practical Nurse Training. In J. Keengwe & P. Bull (Eds.), *Handbook of Research on Transformative Digital Content and Learning Technologies* (pp. 374–392). Hershey, PA: IGI Global. doi:10.4018/978-1-5225-2000-9.ch020

Samra, H. E., Li, A. S., Soh, B., & AlZain, M. A. (2019). A Conceptual Model for Cloud-Based E-Training in Nursing Education. In M. Lytras, L. Daniela, & A. Visvizi (Eds.), *Knowledge-Intensive Economies and Opportunities for Social, Organizational, and Technological Growth* (pp. 295–310). Hershey, PA: IGI Global. doi:10.4018/978-1-5225-7347-0.ch015

Sharma, S., & Mann, N. (2018). Workplace Discrimination: The Most Critical Issue in Managing Diversity. In N. Sharma, V. Singh, & S. Pathak (Eds.), *Management Techniques for a Diverse and Cross-Cultural Workforce* (pp. 206–223). Hershey, PA: IGI Global. doi:10.4018/978-1-5225-4933-8.ch012

Simuth, J. (2017). Psychological Impacts of Downsizing Trauma. In S. Háša & R. Brunet-Thornton (Eds.), *Impact of Organizational Trauma on Workplace Behavior and Performance* (pp. 120–139). Hershey, PA: IGI Global. doi:10.4018/978-1-5225-2021-4.ch005

Singh, G., Singh, P., & Singh, M. (2018). Thinking Globally, Leading Locally: Defining Leadership in Diverse Workforce. In N. Sharma, V. Singh, & S. Pathak (Eds.), *Management Techniques for a Diverse and Cross-Cultural Workforce* (pp. 98–115). Hershey, PA: IGI Global. doi:10.4018/978-1-5225-4933-8.ch006

Singh, S. (2018). Exploring the Relationship Between Organizational Culture and WLB. In N. Sharma, V. Singh, & S. Pathak (Eds.), *Management Techniques for a Diverse and Cross-Cultural Workforce* (pp. 280–296). Hershey, PA: IGI Global. doi:10.4018/978-1-5225-4933-8.ch016

Slagter van Tryon, P. J. (2017). The Nurse Educator's Role in Designing Instruction and Instructional Strategies for Academic and Clinical Settings. In J. Stefaniak (Ed.), *Advancing Medical Education Through Strategic Instructional Design* (pp. 133–149). Hershey, PA: IGI Global. doi:10.4018/978-1-5225-2098-6.ch006

Starr-Glass, D. (2017). The Misappropriation of Organizational Power and Control: Managerial Bullying in the Workplace. In B. Christiansen & H. Chandan (Eds.), *Handbook of Research on Human Factors in Contemporary Workforce Development* (pp. 87–109). Hershey, PA: IGI Global. doi:10.4018/978-1-5225-2568-4.ch004

Swing, V. K. (2017). Early Identification of Transformation in the Proficiency Level of Critical Thinking: In the Associate Degree Nursing Student. In F. Topor (Ed.), *Handbook of Research on Individualism and Identity in the Globalized Digital Age* (pp. 190–211). Hershey, PA: IGI Global. doi:10.4018/978-1-5225-0522-8.ch009

Szymanski, M., & Schindler, E. (2017). Embracing Organizational Trauma: Positive Effects of Death Experiences on Organizational Culture – Three Short Case Studies. In S. Háša & R. Brunet-Thornton (Eds.), *Impact of Organizational Trauma on Workplace Behavior and Performance* (pp. 247–263). Hershey, PA: IGI Global. doi:10.4018/978-1-5225-2021-4.ch010

Tiwari, V., & Singh, S. K. (2017). Relationship Among Work-Related Micro-OB Variables: A Model Approach. In B. Christiansen & H. Chandan (Eds.), *Handbook of Research on Organizational Culture and Diversity in the Modern Workforce* (pp. 261–275). Hershey, PA: IGI Global. doi:10.4018/978-1-5225-2250-8.ch012

Tran, B. (2017). Impact of Organizational Trauma on Workplace Behavior and Performance: Workplace Bullying Due to (In)Competency. In S. Háša, & R. Brunet-Thornton (Eds.), Impact of Organizational Trauma on Workplace Behavior and Performance (pp. 221-245). Hershey, PA: IGI Global. doi:10.4018/978-1-5225-2021-4.ch009

Tran, B. (2017). Organizational Diversity: From Workforce Diversity to Workplace Inclusion for Persons With Disabilities. In B. Christiansen & H. Chandan (Eds.), *Handbook of Research on Organizational Culture and Diversity in the Modern Workforce* (pp. 100–131). Hershey, PA: IGI Global. doi:10.4018/978-1-5225-2250-8.ch006

Uysal, H. T., & Gedik, İ. A. (2017). Effect of Cynical Individual Factor on the Reverse Mobbing Tendency: A Planned Behavior. In B. Christiansen & H. Chandan (Eds.), *Handbook of Research on Organizational Culture and Diversity in the Modern Workforce* (pp. 276–308). Hershey, PA: IGI Global. doi:10.4018/978-1-5225-2250-8.ch013

Wright, V. H., & Davis, A. (2016). Integrating Technology in Nurse Education: Tools for Professional Development, Teaching, and Clinical Experiences. In V. Wang (Ed.), *Handbook of Research on Advancing Health Education through Technology* (pp. 23–38). Hershey, PA: IGI Global. doi:10.4018/978-1-4666-9494-1.ch002

Yuksekdag, B. B. (2017). The Importance of Mobile Augmented Reality in Online Nursing Education. In G. Kurubacak & H. Altinpulluk (Eds.), *Mobile Technologies and Augmented Reality in Open Education* (pp. 291–305). Hershey, PA: IGI Global. doi:10.4018/978-1-5225-2110-5.ch015

Zineldin, M., & Vasicheva, V. (2018). Determinants of Patient Safety and Trust With Focus on Health Care Information Technology (HIT) and Physicians-Nurses Performance. In *Technological Tools for Value-Based Sustainable Relationships in Health: Emerging Research and Opportunities* (pp. 116–126). Hershey, PA: IGI Global. doi:10.4018/978-1-5225-4091-5.ch006

About the Author

Cheryl Green, PhD, DNP, RN, LCSW, CNL, MAC, FAPA is a nurse, and clinical social worker. In nursing, Dr. Green has worked in the areas of medical-surgical nursing, legal nurse consulting, psychiatry, community health, medically-complex rehabilitation, and as a nurse educator. As a social worker, she has had a private practice working with children, families, and couples, worked within private group practices, served as a mental health consultant to a private school, provided spiritually-based therapy in a group practice, and provided play therapy and child-centered family work with children affected and infected with HIV/AIDS at the Yale University Child Study Center in the role of clinical faculty. Dr. Green has also worked as a crisis clinician providing on-call psychiatric consultation within a hospital emergency department setting. Her volunteer work includes: Board member for the Connecticut League of Nursing and executive-at-large, as well as a board member for the Sigma Theta Tau International Nursing Honor Society, Chapter Chi Zeta and Governance Chair. Former American Red Cross health services (and disaster services) volunteer for over 20 years.

Index

P

R

S

T

U

V

W

CPSIA information can be obtained
at www.ICGtesting.com
Printed in the USA
BVHW061722200519
548558BV00006B/56/P

9 781522 573418